EXERCISES IN ORAL RADIOGRAPHY TECHNIQUES
A LABORATORY MANUAL

Third Edition

Evelyn M. Thomson, BSDH, MS
Adjunct Assistant Professor
Gene W. Hirschfeld School of Dental Hygiene
Old Dominion University
Norfolk, Virginia

Pearson

Boston   Columbus   Indianapolis   New York   San Francisco   Upper Saddle River
Amsterdam   Cape Town   Dubai   London   Madrid   Milan   Munich   Paris   Montreal   Toronto
Delhi   Mexico City   Sao Paulo   Sydney   Hong Kong   Seoul   Singapore   Taipei   Tokyo

Publisher: Julie Levin Alexander
Assistant to Publisher: Regina Bruno
Editor-in-Chief: Mark Cohen
Executive Editor: John Goucher
Development Editor: Melissa Kerian
Associate Editor: Nicole Ragonese
Editorial Assistant: Rosalie Hawley
Media Editor: Amy Peltier
Media Product Manager: Lorena Cerisano
Managing Production Editor: Patrick Walsh
Production Liaison: Christina Zingone
Production Editor: Erika Jordan
Manufacturing Manager: Alan Fischer
Design Director: Jayne Conte
Cover Designer: Suzanne Behnke
Director of Marketing: David Gesell
Executive Marketing Manager: Katrin Beacom
Marketing Specialist: Michael Sirinides
Composition: Laserwords
Printer/Binder: Bind-Rite Graphics/Robbinsville
Cover Printer: Lehigh-Phoenix Color/Hagerstown
Cover Image: Dental X-Rays, Ocean Photography/Veer

Notice:
The author and the publisher of this volume have taken care that the information and technical recommendations contained herein are based on research and expert consultation and are accurate and compatible with the standards generally accepted at the time of publication. Nevertheless, as new information becomes available, changes in clinical and technical practices become necessary. The reader is advised to carefully consult manufacturers' instructions and information material for all supplies and equipment before use and to consult with a healthcare professional as necessary. This advice is especially important when using new supplies or equipment for clinical purposes. The author and publisher disclaim all responsibility for any liability, loss, injury, or damage incurred as a consequence, directly or indirectly, of the use and application of any of the contents of this volume.

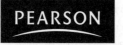

www.pearsonhighered.com

1 2 3 4 5 6 7 8 9 10
ISBN 13: 978-0-13-801944-0
ISBN 10:   0-13-801944-4

Contents

Preface

While dental hygiene and dental assisting students learn oral radiographic theory in the classroom, it is through laboratory practice that these students perfect the skills necessary to assume their professional roles. Currently textbooks are available for students to study oral radiology principles, but there remains a need for a laboratory manual that will challenge students to link theory with clinical practice. The purpose of this book is to provide dental hygiene and dental assisting students with concrete, practical exercises in oral radiographic procedures and interpretation. Designed to complement basic oral radiology theory textbooks, *Exercises in Oral Radiography Techniques: A Laboratory Manual* serves as a workbook to guide the student in the practice of radiographic techniques.

It is the intent of this book to provide students and instructors with ready-made exercises, complete with directions for completing the activity, mounting diagrams to attach the finished radiographs, and pages that allow the student to turn in the assignments for instructor evaluation. Each of the student-driven activities requires minimal preparation by the instructor, and explicit directions guide the student in independent, self-paced practice.

USING THIS MANUAL

Each of the 14 exercises is easily adaptable for use in dental hygiene and dental assisting programs. The exercise modules may be used in any order and are written in a style that allows the instructor to tailor the practice sessions to meet the needs of the program. For example, specific image receptor holding devices may be substituted for those suggested in the exercise. The inclusion of an "Instructor Demonstration" step at the beginning of each module provides an opportunity for the instructor to introduce products, procedures, and protocol that may be particular to that institution.

Students may be directed to copy the mounting pages and continue practicing a technique until mastery, as determined by the instructor, is achieved.

Each exercise begins with an introduction, which provides an overview of the concepts, how the concepts relate to clinical practice, and the rationale for learning the material. Learning objectives are listed for each activity. To evaluate these objectives, study questions are included in each exercise module. Students are challenged to answer the questions based on the outcomes of the activity and/or from reading the material in the key-point outline. The outline following each activity serves as a convenient study guide to accompany a radiology theory textbook. This laboratory manual does not attempt to duplicate theory already covered in depth oral radiology textbooks. The intent of this manual is to complement the basic theory text and be useful to the student as a study guide or as a review of the key concepts.

SUGGESTIONS FOR EDUCATORS

Although the exercises may be used in any order, the instructor may benefit from the sequencing explained here. Laboratory Exercise 1 provides an introduction to radiographic equipment and a film processing and darkroom orientation activity that allows the student to begin the first week of the term or semester with a hands-on laboratory activity, while also including the necessary instruction in the safe operation of dental x-ray equipment. Laboratory Exercise 2 introduces the student to intraoral radiographic techniques with bitewing radiographs. Because many programs are reducing or eliminating film-based radiography, digital imaging technology is introduced in Laboratory Exercise 3. Instructors may choose to implement Laboratory Exercises 2 and 3 simultaneously, allowing the student to begin learning radiographic techniques with digital image receptors. Digital imaging allows the student to immediately observe the results of the technique steps, often with the PID and image receptor still in place. This immediate feedback may provide an advantage over film-based imaging with its possible disconnect between the exposure techniques the student uses and the processing steps required to produce outcomes.

Once introduced to both film-based and digital imaging, the student can progress to learning the periapical radiographic techniques introduced in Laboratory Exercises 4 and 5 and may be directed to complete these exercises either with film or digital technology. Paralleling, the technique of choice for quality imaging, is introduced first in Laboratory Exercise 4. Laboratory Exercise 5 allows the student to gain a working knowledge of the bisecting technique, a skill often used to manage patients unable to tolerate the image receptor placement required for the paralleling technique. Having recently learned and practiced the steps for the paralleling technique in Laboratory Exercise 4, the slight modifications in these steps required for the bisecting technique can be introduced now so that the student can build upon the knowledge he or she has just acquired. However, introducing this laboratory activity just prior to the student practice in Laboratory Exercise 9 Patient Management works as well, especially to prepare the student to alter basic skills learned for the paralleling technique to meet the various needs of patients.

As students produce bitewing and periapical radiographs, they will need to master the skills required for orienting the images with Laboratory Exercise 6 Film Mounting and Radiographic Landmarks. Introducing identification of radiographic anatomy at this point in a typical semester allows educators to take advantage of the probability that students will have acquired a basic knowledge of head and neck anatomy in other coursework that can now be applied to learning how to identify the radiographic appearance of these structures. Having had the opportunity to practice bitewing and periapical techniques, the student should now be able to identify common errors and problem-solve corrective actions in Laboratory Exercise 7 Identifying and Correcting Radiographic Errors.

Having attained this competency level in basic radiographic techniques, the next two exercises facilitate the transfer of these skills from the laboratory setting to a guided pre-clinical student partner practice. To prepare students for this partner practice, infection control protocol for radiographic services is formally introduced in Laboratory Exercise 8. While an instructor may choose to implement this module earlier, placing this activity a few weeks into the term is beneficial in two ways. First, most students will have had the opportunity to learn and practice infection control basics, such as the use of protective barriers and handwashing, in the patient-care pre-clinical course and can now expand on this knowledge to apply infection control methods specifically to the radiographic procedure. Additionally, by this time in a typical semester, the pre-clinical student will have begun to practice instrumentation skills intraorally. When students have had experience maneuvering around the oral cavity, they tend to be more prepared to perform radiographic placement procedures. The initial apprehension that sometimes occurs with the first student partner intraoral practice is eliminated, and the students can concentrate on adapting the radiographic technique skills learned on teaching manikins or skulls to a real-life situation. Laboratory Exercise 9 builds on the initial partner practice by introducing patient management skills required for an apprehensive patient and the patient with a hypersensitive gag reflex, as well as alterations in radiographic techniques required for management of patients with anatomical conditions that interfere with the radiographic technique.

Laboratory Exercises 10, 11, and 12 provide the student with opportunities to learn supplemental techniques, including occlusal and panoramic techniques, and to test tips for acceptable alterations to technique basics that can be used to improve diagnostic quality. Following acquisition of these basic radiographic skills, students should possess an appreciation for producing diagnostic quality radiographs, and Laboratory Exercise 13 will provide an opportunity for students to perform quality control tests. Laboratory Exercise 14 concludes with opportunities for the student to practice the interpretation skills necessary for clinical practice.

ABOUT THE THIRD EDITION

Providing students with guided exercises necessary to obtain dental radiographic skills, while providing instructors of oral radiology with a resource for meaningful laboratory activities, continues to be the goal of this lab manual. Changes were made to the sequencing of the laboratory exercises to better coincide with how the students will use these skills in clinical practice. This sequencing is explained in the previous section *Suggestions for Educators*. Since the last edition, digital imaging has been incorporated more thoroughly into dental hygiene and dental assisting curricula. In fact, many programs now teach digital imaging almost exclusively. In response, each of the laboratory exercises, including panoramic radiography, addresses both film-based and digital imaging. While the laboratory exercise on digital imaging has been updated and expanded, the integration of digital imaging within each of the laboratory modules adds flexibility for educators to use each of the exercises to teach either or both film and digital imaging. Also integrated into the laboratory exercises on bitewing and periapical radiographic techniques are two of the more popular image receptor holding devices, eliminating the need for a separate module on supplemental holders and further adding flexibility for educators to use the exercise activities with their choice of holder.

To meet the American Dental Education Association's Curriculum Guidelines for Allied Dental Education directive that students be provided with basic radiation safety prior to starting laboratory practice, Laboratory Exercise 1 Introduction to Radiation Safety and Dental Radiographic Equipment has been added. Manual processing is no longer the focus of the first exercise, reflecting the reality that the student is not likely to encounter this older technique in practice. Responding further to technological advances, the laboratory exercise on exposure variables has been eliminated based on educators' input that modern dental x-ray equipment is not likely to have variable exposure controls or removable PIDs. Updates to the laboratory exercise on supplemental radiographic techniques include separating out the activities for learning occlusal radiographic techniques into a stand-alone chapter to make room for activities where students can try out real-life tips for both film-based and digital imaging.

ACKNOWLEDGMENTS

Exercises in Oral Radiography Techniques: A Laboratory Manual represents a collection of teaching strategies developed over the years of teaching oral radiology to dental hygiene and dental assisting students and interacting with colleagues. This book would not have been possible without the support and assistance of the students, faculty, and staff at Old Dominion University, Gene W. Hirschfeld School of Dental Hygiene.

A very special note of appreciation goes to my husband Hu Odom for his loving support and encouragement.

Evie

Reviewers

Joanna Campbell, RDH, MA
Bergen Community College
Paramus, New Jersey

Barbara R. Ellis, RDH, MA
Monroe Community College
Rochester, New York

Frances McConaughy, RDH, MS
Weber State University
Ogden, Utah

Ann Prey, RDH, MS
Milwaukee Area Technical College
Milwaukee, Wisconsin

Janice M. Williams, BSDH, MS
Tennessee State University
Nashville, Tennessee

laboratory exercise 1

Introduction to Radiation Safety and Dental Radiographic Equipment

INTRODUCTION

Dental radiographs play a key role in diagnosing and treating dental diseases. Although dental radiographs are often necessary for detection and assessment of oral conditions, their benefit must be balanced with the risk exposure to radiation presents. Most experts agree that the small amount of radiation required to produce dental radiographs is not likely to produce a biological response. However, because of the uncertain risks of even small doses, the oral health care team should understand its ethical responsibility to embrace radiation protection measures, not only for the patient but for oneself and other members of the oral health care team during patient exposures. To operate dental x-ray equipment safely, the radiographer must possess a thorough understanding of the components of the x-ray machine, possess a working knowledge of the x-ray machine control panel, and be able to follow established safety protocols for safe operation of the equipment. The purpose of this laboratory exercise is to familiarize you with the safe use of dental x-ray equipment.

OBJECTIVES

Following completion of this lab activity, you will be able to:

1. Identify and specify the function of the components of an intraoral dental x-ray machine.

2. List and specify the function of each setting/variable on the control panel of an intraoral dental x-ray machine.

3. Demonstrate the safe operation of an intraoral dental x-ray machine following a systematic sequence of steps.

4. Demonstrate safety protocol to protect oneself and other members of the oral health care team during patient exposure.

5. Identify and specify the function of the components of an intraoral film packet.

6. Identify the components of a digital imaging system.

7. Demonstrate proficiency in automatic film processing and/or operation of laser scanning PSP (photostimuable phosphor) plates.

MATERIALS

Student partner

Operatory with an intraoral dental x-ray machine and control panel

Lead/lead equivalent apron with thyroid collar

Three size #2 radiographic film packets or PSP plates or one size #2 digital sensor

Small object of varying thickness of metal or other dense material—seashell or step-wedge (available commercially or see Laboratory Exercise 13, Radiographic Quality Assurance Procedure 13–1 for instructions on making your own), or a metal object—such as a coin or key

PREPARATION

1. Study the chapter outline to prepare for this laboratory exercise. An understanding of the material presented in the outline is required to complete this activity.

2. Instructor demonstration may enhance knowledge of the laboratory exercise.

LABORATORY EXERCISE ACTIVITIES

Part 1: Dental X-ray Machine Components

1. Use Worksheet 1–1: Dental X-ray Machine Components to become familiar with the dental x-ray machine. Using the worksheet as a guide, write out your observations in response to the questions.

2. Draw and label a diagram of the components of the dental x-ray machine that you observed.

Part 2: Safety Protocol

1. Use Worksheet 1–2: Safety Protocol to investigate how safety protocol for this x-ray machine has been established.

2. Together with a student partner, simulate the radiographic procedure:
   a. Seat your partner in the treatment chair.
   b. Adjust the chair to a comfortable height.
   c. Place the lead/lead equivalent apron and thyroid collar protective barrier on the patient.

    d. Extend the x-ray tube head and position the tube head and PID (position indicating device) to direct the x-ray beam to simulate imaging the patient's anterior and left and right posterior regions of the oral cavity.

    e. Demonstrate where to stand during patient exposures that would protect the radiographer from radiation exposure.

Part 3: Demonstration of the Steps for Operating the Dental X-ray Machine

1. With a partner, use Worksheet 1–3: Dental X-ray Machine Operation to demonstrate safe operation of the x-ray machine.

2. Use these guidelines to assess your ability to satisfactorily perform the steps for safe operation of the x-ray machine.

3. Practice these protocols until all steps can be performed at a mastery level.

4. Switch partners and repeat the procedure.

Part 4: Effect of Exposure Time on Radiographic Image Density

1. Obtain three size #2 radiographic film packets or PSP plates or one size #2 digital sensor.

2. Turn the power on to the x-ray machine.

3. Check posted exposure settings for the dental x-ray machine and set for the maxillary central incisor periapical radiograph.

4. Place the first image receptor (either film, PSP plate, or digital sensor) on the dental chair or countertop near the x-ray machine.

5. Place a small object made of varying thickness of material such as a seashell or step-wedge (available commercially or see Laboratory Exercise 13, Radiographic Quality Assurance, Procedure 13–1 for instructions on making your own), or a metal object—such as a coin or key on top of the image receptor. (Figure 1–1 ■)

6. Position the x-ray tube head and PID so that the x-rays will be directed perpendicular to the image receptor. Position the open end of the PID approximately 1 inch above the object that was placed on top of the image receptor.

7. Move to the designated location where you will be protected from the source of radiation.

8. Depress the exposure button and hold it down firmly until the exposure is complete.

9. Set this exposed film/PSP plate aside. If using a digital sensor, save this image and open a new image window to prepare for the second exposure.

10. Next, check the posted exposure settings AND DECREASE THE EXPOSURE TIME BY ONE-HALF. For example, if your posted

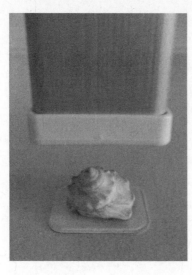

Figure 1–1 Dense object (seashell) placed on top of image receptor (film). Rectangular-shaped PID directed perpendicular to, and 1 inch over, the object and image receptor.

exposure settings chart recommends an exposure time of 16 impulses for proper exposure of the maxillary central incisor periapical radiograph, you would now decrease that exposure time to 8 (16 ÷ 2 = 8).

11. Place the second film packet/PSP plate on the dental chair or countertop near the x-ray machine and place the same object used for the first exposure on top of this second image receptor. If using a digital sensor, there is no need to move the sensor or object between exposures. Use the same setup that was used for the first exposure.

12. Repeat steps 6 through 9 at the decreased exposure time.

13. Next, check the posted exposure settings AND INCREASE THE EXPOSURE TIME BY ONE-HALF. For example, if your posted exposure settings chart recommends an exposure time of 16 impulses for proper exposure of the maxillary central incisor periapical radiograph, you would now increase that exposure time to 24 (16 + 8 = 24).

14. Repeat steps 5 through 8.

15. Follow the steps for automatic processing explained in the outline to process all three films. If using PSP or digital technology, follow the steps explained in the outline for using the laser scanner to obtain the digital images.

16. Observe the resultant images.

COMPETENCY AND EVALUATION

1. Based on your observations of the dental x-ray equipment, describe how the radiographer will be protected during patient exposures.

2. How does knowledge of the dental x-ray machine components contribute to radiation safety? Give examples of how radiation safety may be compromised if the radiographer lacks knowledge of the dental x-ray machine operation.

3. Mount the processed films (now called radiographs) on the simulated film mounts that follow. Secure with a piece of tape placed along the top edge of the radiograph only, so that it may be raised slightly to allow light underneath for ease of viewing. The use of removable transparent tape will allow the film mount page to be used more than once. (If using digital technology, observe the images on the computer monitor or print out a copy of the images at the direction of your instructor.)

4. Examine each of the radiographs. Compare the correctly exposed and the under- and overexposed radiographs and observe any differences in the density (overall darkness or lightness) of the images. Based on your results, what is the effect of altering the exposure time on the radiographic image?

5. Obtain instructor feedback. Identify whether the processing methods were performed correctly.

6. Complete the study questions.

Part 4: Effect of exposure time on radiographic image density

Mount the radiographs below. If using PSP or digital technology, attach a printout of the radiographic images to this page.

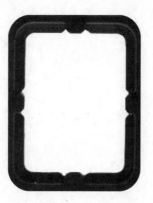

Normal exposure

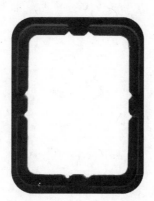

Underexposure

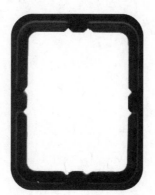

Overexposure

NAME _____

WORKSHEET 1–1: DENTAL X-RAY MACHINE COMPONENTS

The x-ray machine I observed is located in room/cubicle # _____.

Tube head

1. What is the PID (position indicating device) length? (8 inch or 12 inch or 16 inch)

2. What is the PID shape? (round or rectangular)

3. In what direction(s) can the PID be moved?

4. What are the numbers on the tube head yoke for?

5. Set the PID to +20 degrees. In what direction will the x-ray beam be directed toward in this position? (ceiling or floor)

Extension arm

6. Move the tube head from its closed extension arm position into the position toward where the patient will be seated. Does the tube head remain stable in this new position? Reposition the tube head around the dental chair where the patient will be seated. Does the tube head remain stable in each position you place it in?

7. In what direction(s) does the yoke allow the tube head to be moved?

Control panel

8. Where is the unit power or ON/OFF button located?

9. How do you know if the power is on or off?

10. What is the kilovoltage (kVp) setting for this x-ray machine? Can the operator change the kVp setting or has the machine manufacturer preset this variable?

11. What is the milliamperage (mA) setting for this x-ray machine? Can the operator change the mA setting or has the machine manufacturer preset this variable?

12. What is the range of impulse/time settings for this x-ray machine? Can the operator change the impulses/time?

13. When is this dental x-ray machine due for state or local inspection? How would you find out this information?

NAME _____

WORKSHEET 1–2: SAFETY PROTOCOL

1. Where is the exposure button for this dental x-ray machine located?

2. How did you know this exposure button was for this x-ray machine and not a nearby unit?

3. How does the location of the exposure button protect the radiographer during exposure?

4. What barriers are in place to protect other members of the oral health care team during exposure?

5. Is there a recommended distance away from the source of radiation used to protect others who may be in the vicinity of the exposure? What is this distance?

6. How does the radiographer know when an exposure is being activated?

7. How would the radiographer know what settings to use for an anterior or posterior radiograph; or for a child or an adult?

NAME _____

WORKSHEET 1–3: DENTAL X-RAY MACHINE OPERATION

Satisfactorily
Performed
✓

1. Turn the power on. _____

2. Choose to simulate an exposure of a bitewing radiograph
   on an adult patient and, unless these are preset by the
   manufacturer, select the mA and kVp settings that would
   be best suited for the exposure. _____

3. Select the impulse/time setting. _____

4. Utilizing the extension arm and yoke, adjust the tube
   head by aligning the PID so that the central beam of
   radiation is directed down toward the empty dental
   chair. The vertical angulation should be set at approximately
   90 degrees to the dental chair in this position. _____

5. Move to the appropriately protected location from the
   source of radiation. _____

6. Depress the exposure button and hold it down firmly
   until the exposure is complete. The audible signal and
   x-ray exposure indicator light will activate for the duration
   of the exposure. _____

7. When the procedure is complete fold the tube head
   support extension arm into the closed, neutral position. _____

8. Turn off the power to the x-ray machine. _____

I. Dental x-ray machine components (Figure 1–2 ■)
   A. Control panel (Figure 1–3 ■)
      1. Power (ON/OFF) control
      2. Milliamperage (mA) control (may be preset by the unit manufacturer)
         a. Controls the amount of radiation reaching the image receptor
         b. Directly proportional to image density
            1) Increased mA results in increased image density
            2) Decreased mA results in decreased image density
      3. Kilovoltage (kVp) control (may be preset by the unit manufacturer)
         a. Controls the penetrating power of the x-ray beam
         b. Directly proportional to the image density
            1) Increased penetration of the x-ray beam results in more x-ray photons reaching the image receptor.
            2) Decreased penetration of the x-ray beam results in fewer x-ray photons reaching the image receptor.

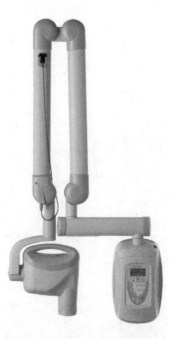

Figure 1–2 Intraoral dental x-ray machine. (Image courtesy of Progeny, a Midmark Company)

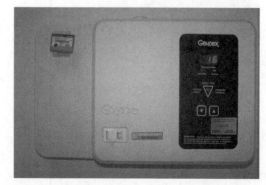

Figure 1–3 Dental x-ray machine control panel and exposure button.

      c. Inversely proportional to the image contrast
        1) Increased penetration of the x-ray beam results in lower image contrast.
        2) Decreased penetration of the x-ray beam results in higher image contrast.
    4. Exposure time (impulses)
      a. Controls the length of time the patient is exposed to the set mA and kVp conditions
      b. Directly proportional to the image density
        1) Increased exposure time results in more x-ray photons reaching the image receptor.
        2) Decreased exposure time results in fewer x-ray photons reaching the image receptor.
    5. Exposure button (may be on the control panel or in a remote location) (Figure 1–4 ■)
      a. The radiographer's finger must engage the exposure switch for the duration of the timer setting or the exposure will terminate.
      b. An audible sound (beep) and an indicator light will activate for the duration of the exposure indicating that radiation is being emitted.
 B. Extension arm and tube head support
    1. These allow the tube head to be moved into position near the patient's oral structures.
    2. A yoke attached to the extension arm allows the tube head to be moved in the vertical (up and down) and the horizontal (side-to-side) directions.

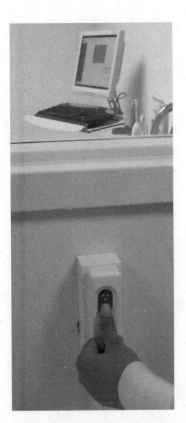

Figure 1–4 Exposure button location that allows the radiographer to remain in a protected area.

C. Tube head
   1. Houses the vacuum tube where x-rays are generated
   2. Provides protection and insulation to the vacuum tube
   3. Is lead lined to prevent stray radiation from escaping
D. PID (positioning indicating device)
   1. Extends from the tube head
   2. Used to direct the x-rays toward the structures to be imaged
   3. Is round cylinder or rectangular shaped
      a. It collimates (restricts) the beam to a specific diameter.
      b. Rectangular-shaped PID reduces the amount of radiation reaching the patient by approximately 70 percent over the round cylinder PID (Figure 1–1).
   4. Available in various lengths: 8 inch, 12 inch, and 16 inch
      a. Long PID may be recessed into the tube head, giving the appearance of being shorter (Figure 1–5 ■).
      b. Long PID projects a less divergent x-ray beam, resulting in less patient radiation exposure.

II. Radiation safety
A. ALARA—As low as reasonably achievable
   1. Concept embraced by the oral health care team
   2. States that efforts should be made to reduce radiation doses whenever feasible
B. Radiographer protection
   1. Time
      a. Limit time spent near x-ray generating equipment.
      b. Avoid errors that result in retake radiographs that increase time spent near x-ray generating equipment.
   2. Shielding
      a. Place structural shielding between operator and source of x-ray generating equipment (Figure 1–4).
      b. 1 millimeter of lead and most building construction materials provide adequate protection. These include plaster, cinderblock, 3 inches of drywall, and 3/16 inch steel.
   3. Distance
      a. If structure shielding is not available, remain a minimum of 6 feet away from the source of radiation.
      b. If structure shielding is not available, take a position 45 degrees to the primary x-ray beam as it exits the patient (Figure 1–6 ■).

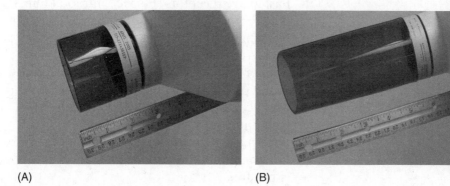

(A)   (B)

Figure 1–5 Comparison of a recessed (A) 8 inch and (B) 12 inch PID. Note the ruler measurement of the PID lengths, indicating that the x-ray tube is located in the back of the tube head.

Radiation Safety and Dental Radiographic Equipment   **17**

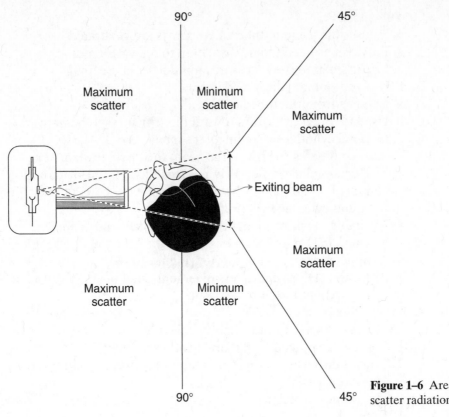

Figure 1–6 Areas of maximum and minimum scatter radiation.

C. Patient protection
  1. Professional judgment
     a. Expose only necessary radiographs.
     b. Use assessment data and evidence-based selection criteria to determine when a patient needs a radiographic examination.
  2. Technical ability of the operator
     a. Communicate with patient to gain cooperation that avoids error that result in retake radiographs.
     b. Evaluate and monitor skills to maintain consistently diagnostic quality results. Obtain continuing education as needed to attain a working knowledge of state-of-the-art procedures as technologies advance the practice of oral radiography.
  3. Equipment standards
     a. Fast image receptors (F-speed intraoral film, PSP plate technology, and digital sensors) require less radiation.
     b. Rectangular collimation reduces radiation exposure 70 percent over round.
     c. Longer length PID (12 or 16 inch) combined with the use of the paralleling technique reduces patient radiation dose when compared with a short PID (8 inch) and the bisecting technique.
     d. Use an image receptor holder and not the patient's finger or thumb to hold the intraoral image receptor in place during exposure.
     e. Place lead/lead equivalent apron and thyroid collar on patient (Figure 1–7 ■).

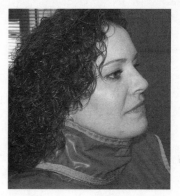

Figure 1–7 Lead apron with thyroid collar.

III. Radiographic film
   A. Intraoral film packet components and function
      1. Film—image receptor (one or two films per packet)
      2. Outer plastic or paper wrap—moisture proof
      3. Black paper—light-tight
      4. Lead foil—absorbs scatter radiation
   B. Intraoral film composition
      1. Base—polyester acetate
      2. Adhesive
      3. Emulsion
         a. Silver halide crystals—light and x-ray sensitive component of the film
         b. Gelatin—suspends and evenly disperses the silver halide crystals
      4. Protective coating
   C. Intraoral film sizes
      1. #0—22 mm × 35 mm—most commonly used for bitewing and periapical radiographs for children with primary dentition
      2. #1—24 mm × 40 mm—most commonly used for bitewing and periapical radiographs for children with primary or mixed primary and permanent dentition; also used for adult vertical bitewing and periapical radiographs of the anterior region
      3. #2—31 mm × 41 mm—most commonly used for adult bitewing (horizontal and vertical) and periapical radiographs; when tolerated, can also be used for bitewing and periapical radiographs on children with mixed primary and permanent dentition; may be substituted for size #4 when exposing occlusal radiographs on children or a localized region on adults
      4. #3—27 mm × 54 mm—specifically designed for adult horizontal bitewings
      5. #4—57 mm × 76 mm—specifically designed for adult occlusal radiographs; when tolerated, can also be used for occlusal radiographs on children with mixed primary and permanent dentition
   D. Intraoral film speeds
      1. D speed is the slowest dental x-ray film currently available, requiring a greater amount of radiation exposure to produce a diagnostic image.

2. E speed requires an estimated one-half the amount of radiation exposure as D-speed film to produce a diagnostic image; while still available from limited manufacturers, E-speed film has been largely replaced by F-speed film.

3. F speed is the fastest dental x-ray film currently available, requiring the least amount of radiation exposure to produce a diagnostic image; estimated to be about 60 percent less exposure than D-speed film to produce a diagnostic image.

IV. Radiographic film processing

    A. Processing methods

        1. Manual processing method

           a. Advantages

             1) Reliable (not subject to equipment malfunction)

             2) Allows operator precise control over time and temperature

             3) If using concentrated or heated chemistry, can be used to produce chairside working radiographs such as those needed during endodontic therapy (root canal operations); called rapid processing

           b. Limitations

             1) Time consuming

             2) Requires manual regulation of solution temperature and manual timing methods

        2. Automatic processing method

           a. Advantages

             1) Increased volume of films may be processed in less time

             2) Automatically regulates time/temperature

           b. Limitations

             1) Possible equipment malfunction

             2) Meticulous maintenance required for optimal output

    B. Processing solutions

        1. Developer

           a. Hydroquinone—reducing agent

           b. Sodium carbonate—activator

           c. Potassium bromide—restrainer

           d. Sodium sulfite—preservative

           e. Distilled water—solvent

        2. Water—removes residual chemistry from film

        3. Fixer

           a. Sodium thiosulfate—clearing agent

           b. Acetic acid—activator

           c. Potassium alum—hardening agent

           d. Sodium sulfite—preservative

           e. Distilled water—solvent

    C. Processing procedures

        1. Manual processing steps

           a. Select film hanger and label to identify films.

           b. Open the light-tight cover of the manual processing tank and stir the developer and fixer solutions to ensure even concentration throughout tank. (Use different stirring paddle for each, developer and fixer, to prevent contamination of solutions.)

           c. Check developer temperature.

    d. Refer to time/temperature recommendations of solution manufacturer, and set timer. (Optimal time/temperature for manually processed radiographs is 68° F for 5 minutes.)

    e. Lock darkroom door, turn off white light, turn on safelight.

    f. Open film packets (recommended infection control procedure for opening film packets is discussed in detail in Laboratory Exercise 8, Infection Control and Student Partner Practice) and place films on hanger.

    g. Immerse films into developer solution and agitate film hanger for 5 seconds to release trapped air bubbles.

    h. Set timer (time dependent on temperature of the developer solution).

    i. Close light-tight cover while film is developing.

    j. When the developing time is complete, under safelight conditions, open the light-tight cover and remove film hanger, with films attached, from developer solution.

    k. Immerse film hanger into water rinse and agitate for 30 seconds.

    l. Immerse film hanger into the fixer solution and agitate film hanger for 5 seconds to release trapped air bubbles.

    m. Activate timer for 10 minutes.

    n. Close light-tight cover for the first 3 minutes of fixation. (It is safe to view the films under white light after 2 or 3 minutes of fixation for a "wet reading," following which the films must be returned to the fixer solution for completion of the 10 minutes of fixation time for archival quality films.)

    o. Remove film hanger from fixer solution when time is up.

    p. Immerse films in water wash for 20 minutes.

    q. Place film hanger in a commercially made film dryer or hang in the air-dry area when wash is complete.

    r. Mount and label dried films (now called radiographs).

  2. Automatic processing steps

    a. Turn on automatic processing machine.

    b. Set appropriate time/temperature as indicated by the manufacturer's instructions.

    c. Lock darkroom door, turn off white light, turn on safelight.

    d. Open film packets (recommended infection control procedure for opening film packets is discussed in detail in Laboratory Exercise 8, Infection Control and Student Partner Practice) and place films into automatic processor.

    e. Allow rollers to take film before releasing.

    f. Wait 10 seconds before placing an additional film into slot to avoid overlapping films.

    g. Retrieve processed films (now called radiographs) when cycle is complete.

    h. Mount and label the radiographs.

V. Digital image receptors

  A. Photostimuable phosphor (PSP); also called storage phosphor system

    1. Digital plate coated with a phosphor (europium activated barium fluorohalide) acts similar to silver halide crystals in conventional film to capture radiation and produce a latent image.

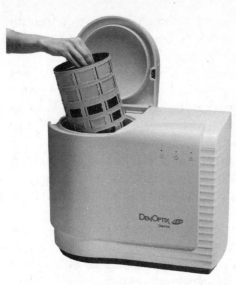

Figure 1–8 Exposed phosphor plates being placed into a laser scanning device. (Courtesy of Gendex Dental Systems)

2. After exposure, the phosphor plate is placed into a laser scanning device (Figure 1–8 ■) that converts the analog data into digital values that the computer reconstructs as an image on a monitor.
3. PSP plates are available in dimensions similar to film sizes #0, #1, #2, #3, and #4.
4. The same holders and biteblocks used for positioning intraoral film can usually be used to position PSP plates.
5. Referred to as indirect digital imaging technology because the laser scanning step required after exposure is considered a "developing" step similar to film-based radiography.
6. Exposure steps
    a. Wipe the PSP plate with an intermediate-level disinfectant and cover with appropriate infection control barrier (see Laboratory Exercise 8, Infection Control and Student Partner Practice).
    b. Place into image receptor holder, position intraorally, and expose.
    c. Remove the PSP plate from the oral cavity, remove the plastic barrier, and disinfect according to manufacturer's instructions. If exposing additional PSP plates, keep exposed plates protected from bright light.
    d. Place exposed PSP plates into laser scanner and activate.
    e. Observe images on computer monitor.
    f. The scanning process may include an erase feature. If not, erase PSP plates by exposing to bright light for the time recommended by manufacturer so that they can be reused.
B. Solid state sensor (CCD: charge-coupled device or CMOS: complementary metal oxide technology)
    1. Electronic chip encased in the sensor converts x-rays into an electronic signal that is sent to the computer via a wire or wirelessly through radio frequency.
    2. Sensors are available in dimensions similar to film sizes #0, #1, and #2.

3. Usually require holders and biteblocks specifically designed for digital sensors and will vary depending on the manufacturer.
4. Referred to as direct digital imaging because radiographic image may be viewed on a computer monitor almost immediately after exposure.
5. Exposure steps
   a. Wipe the sensor with an intermediate-level disinfectant and cover with appropriate infection control barrier (see Laboratory Exercise 8, Infection Control and Student Partner Practice).
   b. Place into image receptor holder, position intraorally, and expose.
   c. Observe the image on the computer monitor to determine diagnostic quality. If retake needed, reposition the sensor without completely removing from the oral cavity.
   d. When examination is complete, remove the sensor from the oral cavity, remove the plastic barrier, and disinfect according to manufacturer's instructions.

VI. Visual characteristics of the radiographic image
   A. Density
      1. This is defined as the overall darkness of the image.
      2. It is related to the amount of radiation reaching the image receptor.
      3. Decreasing the mA exposure setting and/or the exposure time decreases the radiographic image density.
      4. Increasing the mA exposure setting and/or the exposure time increases the radiographic image density.
   B. Contrast (Figure 1–9 ■)
      1. Differences in densities between various regions of the image
      2. High contrast
         a. Very dark areas and very light areas, little shade gradient in between
         b. Also referred to as short scale
         c. Decreasing the kVp exposure setting increases the contrast.

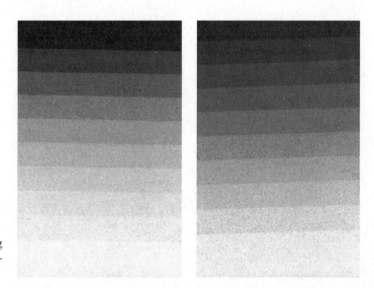

Figure 1–9 Exposure of a step-wedge (varying thickness of metal bands) showing high contrast (left) and low contrast (right).

3. Low contrast
   a. Relatively dark and light areas, with many shade gradients in between
   b. Also referred to as long scale
   c. Increasing the kVp exposure setting decreases the contrast.
C. Radiopaque
   1. Light gray to white or clear areas of the image
   2. Represents dense objects not easily penetrated by the x-ray beam
D. Radiolucent
   1. Dark gray to black areas of the image
   2. Represents less dense objects easily penetrated by the x-ray beam

REFERENCES

American Dental Association Council on Scientific Affairs. (2006). The use of dental radiographs: Update and recommendations. *J. Am. Dent. Assn.*, 137, 1304–1312.

Carestream Health Inc. (2008). *Exposure and processing for dental film radiography.* Rochester, NY, 2007, N-413 CAT No. 832 8783.

Darby, M. L. (2011). *Mosby's comprehensive review of dental hygiene* (7th ed.). St. Louis, MO: Mosby/Elsevier.

Horner, K., Drage, N., & Brettle, D. (2008). *21st century imaging.* London: Quintessence Publishing Co., Ltd.

Thomson, E. M. (2006). Radiation safety update. *Contemp Oral Hyg.* 6(3), 10–18.

Thomson, E. M., & Johnson, O. N. (2012). *Essentials of dental radiography for dental assistants and hygienists* (9th ed.). Upper Saddle River, NJ: Pearson.

1. Which of the following intraoral dental x-ray machine components is used to aim and direct the x-ray beam toward image receptor?
   A. Position indicating device
   B. Extension arm
   C. Control panel
   D. Yoke

2. Where is the ON/OFF switch of an intraoral dental x-ray machine located?
   A. Position indicating device
   B. Extension arm
   C. Control panel
   D. Yoke

3. Which of the following is NOT an exposure variable setting for the dental x-ray machine?
   A. Milliamperage
   B. Kilovoltage
   C. Impulse/exposure time
   D. Density/contrast

4. Each of the following will help to protect the radiographer while operating a dental x-ray machine EXCEPT one. Which one is the EXCEPTION?
   A. Remain behind a structural barrier such as a wall.
   B. Release the exposure button immediately upon hearing the audible beep.
   C. If the x-ray machine is in an open setting, take a position 6 feet away.
   D. Avoid retake radiographs that increase the amount of time spent near the x-ray machine.

5. Each of the following will help limit or reduce radiation exposure to the patient EXCEPT one. Which one is the EXCEPTION?
   A. Fast speed image receptors such as F-speed film and digital sensors
   B. Evidence-based selection criteria that determine need for radiographs
   C. Short (8 inch) position-indicating device combined with the bisecting technique
   D. Rectangular collimation and image receptor holders

6. Which of the following provides a moisture-resistant barrier for an intraoral film?
   A. Plastic/paper wrap
   B. Black paper
   C. Lead foil
   D. Gelatin

7. The undeveloped and unexposed silver halide crystals are removed from the emulsion by
   A. Acetic acid
   B. Hydroquinone
   C. Potassium alum
   D. Sodium thiosulfate
   E. Water

8. Solid state sensors (CCD: charge-coupled device or CMOS: complementary metal oxide technology) require the use of each of the following EXCEPT one. Which one is the EXCEPTION?
   A. Dental x-ray machine
   B. Computer
   C. Laser scanner
   D. Monitor

9. Provided Part 4: "Effect of exposure time on radiographic image density" of this laboratory exercise was performed correctly, there should be a difference in density (overall darkness/lightness) between the three radiographs obtained in the experiment. Which radiograph is darkest?
   A. The first radiograph exposed at the posted exposure settings
   B. The second radiograph exposed at the decreased exposure settings
   C. The third radiograph exposed at the increased exposure settings

10. Based on the outcomes of the exercise performed in Part 4: "Effect of exposure time on radiographic image density," what is your conclusion regarding varying the exposure time?
    A. Image density is inversely proportional to the exposure time.
    B. Image density is directly proportional to the exposure time.

Bitewing Radiographic Technique

INTRODUCTION

Bitewing radiographs play an important role in detecting proximal surface (between the teeth) caries (dental decay) and imaging the supporting bone levels important in the evaluation of periodontal diseases. Using a size #0, #1, #2, or #3 image receptor (either film or photostimuable [PSP] plate or digital sensor), bitewing radiographs image the coronal portion of both the maxillary and the mandibular teeth. When exposing bitewing radiographs, the intraoral image receptor has traditionally been placed in the mouth with the longer dimension positioned horizontally. In fact, the size #3 image receptor is specifically designed for exposing horizontal bitewing radiographs on adult patients (Figure 2–1 ■). However, a vertical placement of the image receptor has been found to be more useful when the focus is on the periodontium or root caries (Figure 2–2 ■). Vertical bitewing radiographs increase the amount of information recorded in the vertical direction. In cases of advanced periodontal disease, the full extent of alveolar bone resorption may not be fully imaged on the horizontally placed bitewing radiograph. Whether positioned horizontally or vertically, precise angulation and meticulous attention to technique is needed to ensure quality diagnostic bitewing radiographs. Even seemingly minor errors can render a bitewing radiograph undiagnostic.

This laboratory exercise is designed to introduce horizontal and vertical bitewing radiographic techniques. The seemingly complex principles of image geometry involved in exposing bitewing radiographs have been organized into four basic steps. By simplifying the bitewing radiographic technique into

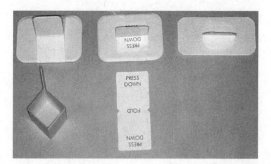

Figure 2–1 Bite loop (left); stick-on tab (center); bitetab pre-attached by the manufacturer to a size #3 film packet designed to be used to expose horizontal bitewing radiographs (right).

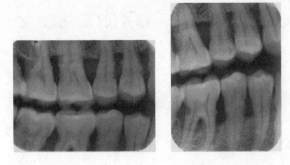

Figure 2–2 A comparison of the image achieved with a horizontally placed image receptor (left) and a vertically placed image receptor (right).

these four basic steps—packet placement, vertical angulation, horizontal angulation, and centering the x-ray beam—the process of producing bitewing radiographs and evaluating the accuracy of technique can be easily mastered. Evaluation of the radiographic image is easier when errors can be attributed to a specific step. Identification of which step is the cause of an error will help pinpoint which skill needs concentrated practice efforts. The simulated mount pages provided in this laboratory exercise may be copied to increase the number of practice sessions required to master the techniques.

There are a variety of commercially made film and digital sensor holding devices on the market. This beginning exercise uses a paper bitewing stick-on tab holder for film-based radiography (Figure 2–3 ■). Similar plastic stick-on tabs are available for digital sensors (Figure 2–4 ■). The use of these types of holders requires a working knowledge of appropriate angles. Mastering these skills with an understanding of projection geometry will allow you to easily transfer this working knowledge to other bitewing image receptor holding devices such as the one noted in Figure 2–5 ■.

OBJECTIVES

Following completion of this lab activity, you will be able to:

1. Demonstrate proficiency in placing, exposing, and processing bitewing radiographs.

2. Correctly identify positive and negative vertical angulation of the PID (position indicating device)

3. Critique a bitewing series for correct (a) placement of the image receptor intraorally; (b) vertical and (c) horizontal angulation of the PID; and (d) exposure by centering the image receptor within the diameter of the x-ray beam.

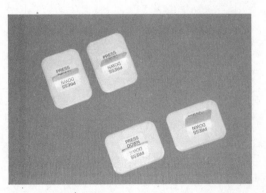

Figure 2–3 Paper bitewing stick-on tabs placed for vertical (top left) and horizontal (bottom right) bitewing radiographs.

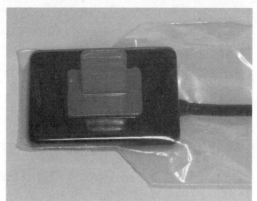

Figure 2–4 Plastic bitewing stick-on tab placed for horizontal bitewing radiographs using a digital sensor.

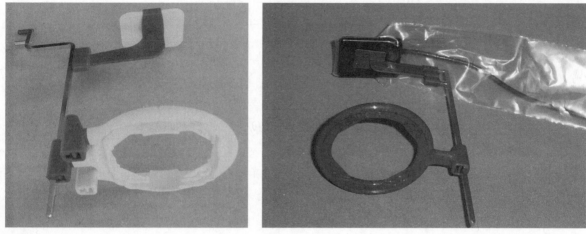

(A)   (B)

Figure 2–5 (A) Film-based and (B) digital sensor bitewing image receptor holders with external aiming device.

MATERIALS

Teaching manikin or skull

Lead/lead equivalent apron with thyroid collar

Size #1, #2, and #3 radiographic films (or photostimuable phosphor [PSP] plates or digital sensors)

Bitewing image receptor holding device (stick-on tab—paper/plastic/foam type or optional holder with external aiming device)

View box

Tongue blades

PREPARATION

1. Study the chapter outline to prepare for this laboratory exercise. An understanding of the material presented in the outline is required to complete this activity.

2. Use Table 2–1 to assist you with completing the exercises. Instructor demonstration may enhance knowledge of the laboratory exercise.

3. Prepare radiology operatory. Set up teaching manikin or skull. Ensure that correct "patient" positioning is achieved, i.e., occlusal plane parallel to the floor, midsagittal plane perpendicular to the floor.

4. Place lead/lead equivalent barrier and thyroid collar over the "patient."

LABORATORY EXERCISE ACTIVITIES

Part 1: Horizontal Bitewing

1. Obtain four size #2 radiographic film packets. (If using digital technology, substitute four size #2 photostimuable phosphor [PSP] plates or one digital sensor for the film packets.)

2. Attach holder to image receptor.

3. Check posted exposure settings for the dental x-ray machine and set for bitewing radiographs.

4. Place and expose the series of bitewing radiographs in the following order:

    1st   right premolar bitewing

    2nd   right molar bitewing

    3rd   left premolar bitewing

    4th   left molar bitewing

    Note: Left-handed radiographers may use this order:

    1st   left premolar bitewing

    2nd   left molar bitewing

    3rd   right premolar bitewing

    4th   right molar bitewing

5. Process the four films or scan the PSP plates or observe the digital images on computer monitor.

Part 2: Horizontal Bitewing Using a Size #3 Film

1. Obtain two size #3 radiographic film packets. (If using digital technology, substitute two size #3 photostimuable phosphor [PSP] plates. Digital sensors are not currently available in size #3.)

2. If not already preattached by the manufacturer, attach the holder to the image receptor (Figure 2–1).

3. Check posted exposure settings for the dental x-ray machine and set for bitewing radiographs.

4. Place and expose the bitewing radiographs in the following order:

    1st   right premolar-molar bitewing

    2nd   left premolar-molar bitewing

TABLE 2–1 Summary of Steps for Acquiring Bitewing Radiographs for Adult Patients

Bitewing Radiograph	Packet Placement	Vertical Angulation	Horizontal Angulation	Centering (direct the central ray of x-ray beam to this point of entry)
Central-Lateral Incisors Image receptor size #1 or size #2 (vertical position)	Center the image receptor to line up behind the right and left central and lateral incisors (Figure 2–6 ■)	+10	Direct the central rays perpendicularly through the left and right central incisor embrasure (Figure 2–7 ■)	A spot on the incisal plane between the maxillary and mandibular central incisors
Canine Image receptor size #1 or size #2 (vertical position)	Center the image receptor to line up behind the canine; include the distal half of the lateral incisor and the mesial half of the first premolar (Figure 2–6)	+10	Direct the central rays perpendicularly at the center of the canine (Figure 2–7)	A spot on the incisal plane between the maxillary and mandibular canines
Premolar Image receptor size #2 (horizontal or vertical position)	Align the anterior edge of the image receptor to line up behind the distal half of the maxillary or the mandibular canine; select the most anteriorly located canine (Figure 2–6)	+10	Direct the central rays perpendicularly through the first and second premolar embrasure (Figure 2–7)	A spot on the occlusal plane between the maxillary and mandibular second premolars
Molar Image receptor size #2 (horizontal or vertical position)	Align the anterior edge of the image receptor to line up behind the distal half of the maxillary or the mandibular second premolar; select the most anteriorly located premolar (Figure 2–6)	+10	Direct the central rays perpendicularly through the first and second molar embrasure (Figure 2–7)	A spot on the occlusal plane between the maxillary and mandibular first molars
Premolar-Molar Image receptor size #3 (horizontal position)	Align the anterior edge of image receptor to line up behind the distal half of the maxillary or the mandibular canine; select the most anteriorly located canine (Figure 2–6)	+10	Direct the central rays perpendicularly through the second premolar and first molar embrasure (Figure 2–7)	A spot on the occlusal plane between the maxillary and mandibular second premolars and the maxillary and mandibular first molars

Reference: Thomson, E. M., & Johnson, O. N. (2012). *Essentials of dental radiography for dental assistants and hygienists* (9th ed.). Upper Saddle River, NJ: Pearson.

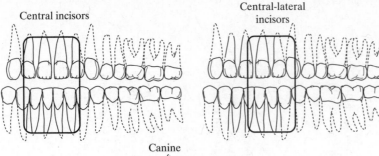

Central incisors

Central-lateral incisors

Canine

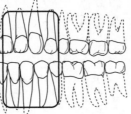

Premolar

Molar

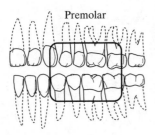

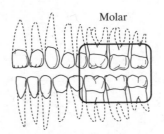

Figure 2–6 Image receptor placement for bitewing radiographs when imaging the central incisors, central-lateral incisors, canines, premolars, and molars bitewing radiographs.

Note: Left-handed radiographers may use this order:

1st   left premolar-molar bitewing

2nd   right premolar-molar bitewing

5. Process the two films or scan the PSP plates.

Part 3: Vertical Bitewing

1. Obtain four size #2 and three size #1 radiographic film packets. (If using digital technology, substitute four size #2 and three size #1 photostimuable phosphor [PSP] plates or one each size #2 and size #1 digital sensor for the film packets.)

2. Attach holder to image receptor. Note: Two stick-on tab holders (paper type) may be placed on anterior bitewing image receptors to aid in placement in the anterior region. (Figure 2–8 ■)

3. Check posted exposure settings for the dental x-ray machine and set for bitewing radiographs.

4. Place and expose the bitewing radiographs in the following order:

1st   central-lateral incisors bitewing

2nd   left canine bitewing

3rd   right canine bitewing

4th   right premolar bitewing

5th   right molar bitewing

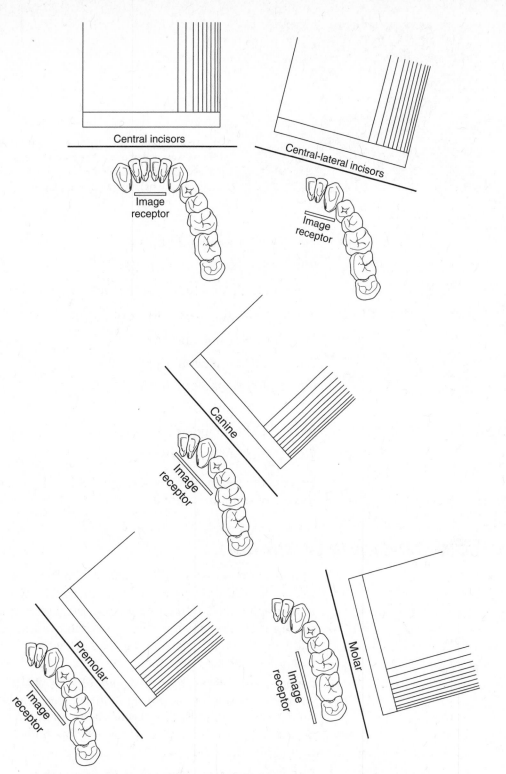

Figure 2–7 Horizontal angulation for bitewing radiographs when imaging the central incisors, central-lateral incisors, canines, premolars, and molars bitewing radiographs can be determined by aligning the open end of the PID parallel to the image receptor. Note the line drawn to indicate that the open end of the PID is parallel to the facial surfaces of the teeth of interest. This line may be visualized through the use of a tongue blade or the external aiming ring of the image receptor holder.

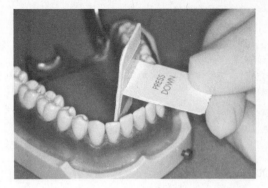

Figure 2–8 Using two stick-on tab bitewing film holders aids in film packet placement in the anterior region by extending the bite surface, allowing placement of the film packet well into the oral cavity where palatal height is greatest.

6th   left premolar bitewing

7th   left molar bitewing

Note: Left-handed radiographers may use this order:

1st   central-lateral incisors bitewing

2nd   right canine bitewing

3rd   left canine bitewing

4th   left premolar bitewing

5th   left molar bitewing

6th   right premolar bitewing

7th   right molar bitewing

5. Process the seven films or scan the PSP plates or observe the digital images on computer monitor.

COMPETENCY AND EVALUATION

1. Mount the processed radiographs on the simulated film mounts that follow. Secure with a piece of tape placed along the top edge of the radiograph only, so that it may be raised slightly to allow light underneath for ease of viewing. The use of removable transparent tape will allow the film mount page to be used more than once. (If using digital technology, observe the images on the computer monitor or print out a copy of the images at the direction of your instructor.)

   Note: Use the labial mounting method. (See Laboratory Exercise 6, Film Mounting and Radiographic Landmarks, for details.) The raised portion of the embossed dot is toward you (convex) when placing the radiograph onto the page.

2. Place the page with the mounted radiographs taped to it on a view box and evaluate for acceptability. Circle the ✓ where packet placement, vertical angulation, horizontal angulation, and centering were performed correctly, and the ✗ where performed incorrectly. Identify which error was made by placing an ✗ on the corresponding line.

3. Obtain instructor feedback. Identify which step (packet placement, vertical angulation, horizontal angulation, centering) needs improvement.

4. Repeat Part 1, Part 2, and/or Part 3 at the direction of your instructor. The film mount page may be copied to accommodate multiple practice attempts to achieve competency.

5. Compare the sets of bitewings with each other. Evaluate the images for diagnostic quality differences and discuss which type (horizontal or vertical) and which size image receptor produced the best images. Why? Assess your skills with each of the techniques. Did you find one or the other technique easier to place into position? Why? Discuss what type of oral conditions would be assessed for horizontal bitewings and for vertical bitewings. What did you discover to be advantages and limitations of each of the skills you learned by completing this exercise?

6. Complete the study questions.

patient's left

Part 1: Horizontal Bitewing Radiographs
Mount Films Below

patient's right

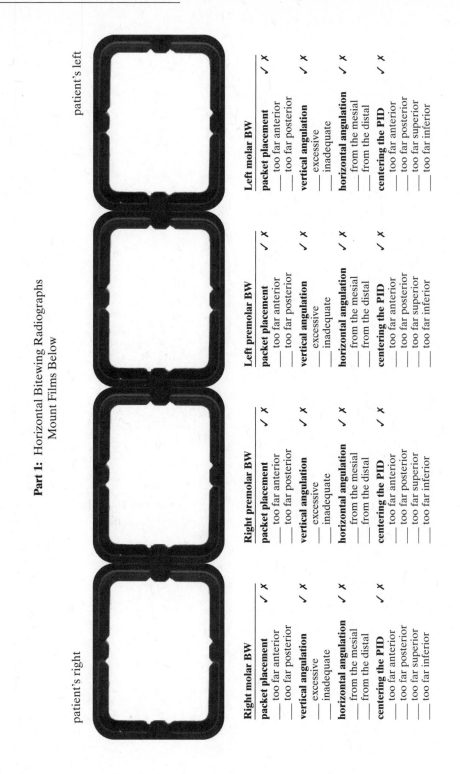

Right molar BW   ✓ ✗

packet placement
___ too far anterior
___ too far posterior

vertical angulation
___ excessive
___ inadequate

horizontal angulation
___ from the mesial
___ from the distal

centering the PID
___ too far anterior
___ too far posterior
___ too far superior
___ too far inferior

Right premolar BW   ✓ ✗

packet placement
___ too far anterior
___ too far posterior

vertical angulation
___ excessive
___ inadequate

horizontal angulation
___ from the mesial
___ from the distal

centering the PID
___ too far anterior
___ too far posterior
___ too far superior
___ too far inferior

Left premolar BW   ✓ ✗

packet placement
___ too far anterior
___ too far posterior

vertical angulation
___ excessive
___ inadequate

horizontal angulation
___ from the mesial
___ from the distal

centering the PID
___ too far anterior
___ too far posterior
___ too far superior
___ too far inferior

Left molar BW   ✓ ✗

packet placement
___ too far anterior
___ too far posterior

vertical angulation
___ excessive
___ inadequate

horizontal angulation
___ from the mesial
___ from the distal

centering the PID
___ too far anterior
___ too far posterior
___ too far superior
___ too far inferior

Part 2: Horizontal Bitewing Radiographs—Utilizing a Size #3 Film
Mount Films Below

patient's right   patient's left

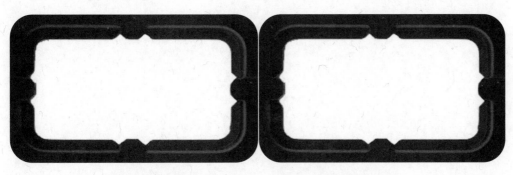

Right molar-premolar BW		**Left molar-premolar BW**	
packet placement	✓ ✗	**packet placement**	✓ ✗
___ too far anterior		___ too far anterior	
___ too far posterior		___ too far posterior	
vertical angulation	✓ ✗	**vertical angulation**	✓ ✗
___ excessive		___ excessive	
___ inadequate		___ inadequate	
horizontal angulation	✓ ✗	**horizontal angulation**	✓ ✗
___ from the mesial		___ from the mesial	
___ from the distal		___ from the distal	
centering the PID	✓ ✗	**centering the PID**	✓ ✗
___ too far anterior		___ too far anterior	
___ too far posterior		___ too far posterior	
___ too far superior		___ too far superior	
___ too far inferior		___ too far inferior	

Part 3: Vertical Bitewing Radiographs
Mount Films Below

patient's left

patient's right

Right molar BW

packet placement ✓ ✗
___ too far anterior
___ too far posterior

vertical angulation ✓ ✗
___ excessive
___ inadequate

horizontal angulation ✓ ✗
___ from the mesial
___ from the distal

centering the PID ✓ ✗
___ too far anterior
___ too far posterior
___ too far superior
___ too far inferior

Right premolar BW

packet placement ✓ ✗
___ too far anterior
___ too far posterior

vertical angulation ✓ ✗
___ excessive
___ inadequate

horizontal angulation ✓ ✗
___ from the mesial
___ from the distal

centering the PID ✓ ✗
___ too far anterior
___ too far posterior
___ too far superior
___ too far inferior

Right canine BW

packet placement ✓ ✗
___ too far anterior
___ too far posterior

vertical angulation ✓ ✗
___ excessive
___ inadequate

horizontal angulation ✓ ✗
___ from the mesial
___ from the distal

centering the PID ✓ ✗
___ too far anterior
___ too far posterior
___ too far superior
___ too far inferior

Central lateral-incisors BW

packet placement ✓ ✗
___ too far anterior
___ too far posterior

vertical angulation ✓ ✗
___ excessive
___ inadequate

horizontal angulation ✓ ✗
___ from the mesial
___ from the distal

centering the PID ✓ ✗
___ too far anterior
___ too far posterior
___ too far superior
___ too far inferior

Left canine BW

packet placement ✓ ✗
___ too far anterior
___ too far posterior

vertical angulation ✓ ✗
___ excessive
___ inadequate

horizontal angulation ✓ ✗
___ from the mesial
___ from the distal

centering the PID ✓ ✗
___ too far anterior
___ too far posterior
___ too far superior
___ too far inferior

Left premolar BW

packet placement ✓ ✗
___ too far anterior
___ too far posterior

vertical angulation ✓ ✗
___ excessive
___ inadequate

horizontal angulation ✓ ✗
___ from the mesial
___ from the distal

centering the PID ✓ ✗
___ too far anterior
___ too far posterior
___ too far superior
___ too far inferior

Left molar BW

packet placement ✓ ✗
___ too far anterior
___ too far posterior

vertical angulation ✓ ✗
___ excessive
___ inadequate

horizontal angulation ✓ ✗
___ from the mesial
___ from the distal

centering the PID ✓ ✗
___ too far anterior
___ too far posterior
___ too far superior
___ too far inferior

I. Bitewing radiographs
- A. Uses
  1. Imaging proximal surfaces
  2. Imaging crestal bone
  3. Caries detection
  4. Imaging defective restorations
  5. Documenting periodontal status
  6. Determining the presence of contributing factors for periodontal disease: calculus, overhanging restorations
- B. Types
  1. Horizontal (Figure 2–2)
     a. Image receptor placed in the mouth with the long dimension positioned horizontally
     b. Considered the traditional bitewing image receptor placement
  2. Vertical (Figure 2–2)
     a. Image receptor placed in the mouth with the long dimension positioned vertically
     b. Increased coverage of the teeth roots and the surrounding periodontium
     c. Particularly useful for imaging root caries and when bone resorption is extensive
     d. Position used for exposure of the anterior region
- C. Image receptor sizes that can be used to expose bitewing radiographs
  1. Size #0
     a. Recommended for children with primary dentition
     b. Suitable for primary dentition with minimal caries activity
     c. Height dimension of the image receptor limits imaging pulp status when extensive caries are present
  2. Size #1
     a. Recommended for children with primary dentition
     b. Slightly larger recording dimensions will provide more diagnostic information
     c. Often used to expose vertical bitewings in the anterior region of adult patients
  3. Size #2
     a. Most common image receptor size for exposing bitewing radiographs
     b. Suitable for children in transitional (mixed primary and permanent) dental state and most all adults
     c. Provides additional information about developing permanent teeth in the child patient
     d. Can be used to expose horizontal or vertical bitewings
  4. Size #3
     a. Specifically designed for the exposure of bitewing radiographs
     b. May not be used to expose vertical bitewing radiographs, especially if manufacturer has preattached the bite tab in the horizontal position

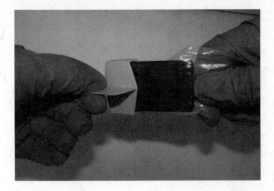

Figure 2–9 Plastic bitewing loop being placed for horizontal bitewing radiographs using a digital sensor.

  c. Longer length records all contact areas of one side of the oral cavity on one image

  d. Allows for the exposure of only two bitewing radiographs in a series: right premolar-molar and left premolar-molar

  e. Limited ability to clearly image all contacts because the premolar and molar regions of the oral cavity are not usually on the same horizontal plane

  f. Shorter height (only 27 mm compared with film size #2, which is 31 mm) may not be suitable for imaging interproximal alveolar bone, especially when bone loss is evident.

 D. Image receptor holders

  1. Designed to hold the image receptor in position to image the crowns of both the maxillary and the mandibular teeth

  2. Examples of bitewing holders

   a. Stick-on bite tabs made of paper, plastic, or foam; may be pre-attached by the manufacturer (Figures 2–1 and 2–4)

   b. Bite loops (Figures 2–1 and 2–9 ■)

   c. Biteblocks with external aiming arm and ring (Figures 2–5)

 E. Principal concepts

  1. White, unprinted side of the film packet positioned toward the teeth. Photostimuable phosphor (PSP) plates are labeled to determine front and back sides. The front side of a digital sensor is flat. If using a wired sensor, the wire is attached to the back.

  2. Image receptor is placed perpendicular to the embrasures (spaces between the teeth) of the maxillary and mandibular teeth of interest. This position will usually also position the image receptor parallel to the facial surfaces of these teeth of interest.

  3. The central ray of the x-ray beam is directed perpendicular to the image receptor through the embrasures, between the teeth of interest.

  4. The image receptor is held in place by a bite tab or other bitewing image receptor holding device.

II. Bitewing radiographic procedure—see Table 2–1

 A. Placement of the image receptor

  1. Place horizontally or vertically depending on regions of interest and patient assessment of need.

  2. Ensure that the image receptor is placed such that a portion of both the maxillary and mandibular teeth of interest will be recorded (Figure 2–10 ■).

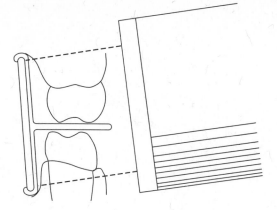

Figure 2–10 Bitewing image receptor position and PID alignment at +10 degrees for recording a portion of both the maxillary and mandibular teeth and crestal bone on the radiograph. Note that the image receptor is centered within the x-ray beam.

3. Vertical placement of the image receptor may not be wide enough to record as many teeth and contact points as horizontal placement.

4. Examine the posterior teeth with the patient occluding to determine which canine and which first premolar, either maxillary or mandibular, is located further anteriorly.

 a. Position the image receptor to align behind the more anteriorly located tooth.

 b. As a general rule, the mandibular canine and the mandibular first premolar will be located further anterior in Class I and Class III occlusion, and the maxillary canine and the maxillary first premolar will be located further anterior in Class II occlusion.

 c. Check both the right and left sides as occlusion can vary.

B. Vertical angulation of the x-ray beam

1. Determine the positive vertical angulation. Positive angulation is achieved by pointing the PID down toward the floor.

2. Using the guide on the tube head, set the positive angulation to approximately +10 degrees for exposure of all posterior and anterior, horizontal and vertical bitewing radiographs on adult patients and to +5 degrees for bitewing radiographs on children who present with primary dentition (Figure 2–11 ■). If no tube head guide is present, vertical angulation is determined by using the floor as a reference point. When the PID is aligned parallel to the floor, the angulation is set at zero. When the PID is directed perpendicular to the floor, the angulation is set at 90 degrees. To

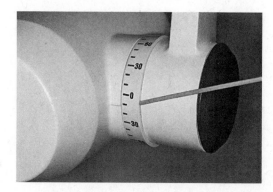

Figure 2–11 Using the guide on the tube head to determine vertical angulation.

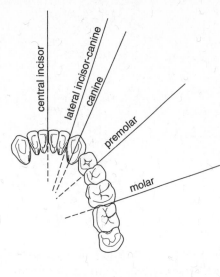

Figure 2–12 Horizontal angulation for bitewing radiographs when imaging the central incisors, central-lateral incisors, canine, premolar, and molar can be determined by directing the central ray of the x-ray beam between a predetermined interproximal space.

set the vertical angulation to +10 degrees, an estimate is made between these two easily identified points (Figure 2–10).

C. Horizontal angulation of the x-ray beam

    1. Determine the side-to-side placement of the PID.

    2. Align the PID such that the central ray of the x-ray beam will intersect the image receptor perpendicularly. Perpendicular alignment of the beam can be achieved either of two ways:

      a. Direct the central ray of the x-ray beam through a predetermined interproximal space (Figure 2–12 ■). Examine the contact points of the patient's teeth to determine the correct angulation for aiming the central ray. Because of the larger size and rhomboid shape of the maxillary posterior teeth, it is helpful to use the maxillary teeth when determining the correct horizontal angulation for posterior bitewing radiographs.

      b. Using the open end of the PID as the reference point, align the PID such that the open end of the PID is parallel to the image receptor in the horizontal plane (Figure 2–7). Visualizing the horizontal placement of the PID is easily achieved by using an image receptor holder with an external aiming device (Figure 2–13 ■) or by placing a tongue blade or cotton-tipped applicator across the open end and rotating the tube head horizontally until the tongue blade or cotton-tipped applicator, and therefore the open end of the PID, is parallel to the image receptor (Figure 2–14 ■).

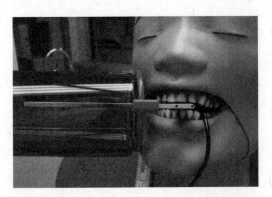

Figure 2–13 Using an image receptor holder with an external aiming ring to visualize correct horizontal angulation.

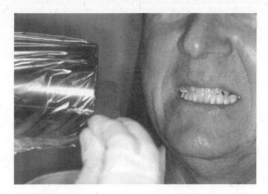

Figure 2–14 Using a tongue blade to visualize correct horizontal angulation.

D. Centering the image receptor within the diameter of the x-ray beam
   1. Determine the placement of the image receptor. Use any part of the image receptor holder that is visible outside the mouth as an indication of where the image receptor is located (Figure 2–13).
   2. Using the bite tab holder as a reference point, align the PID directly over the image receptor (Figure 2–10). The tab should appear to be centered within the diameter of the extending tongue blade (Figure 2–15 ■).

III. Errors
   A. Image receptor placement error
      1. Occurs when the image receptor is not placed correctly in relationship to the teeth of interest
      2. Results in the appropriate teeth not being recorded on the image receptor
      3. Placed too far anteriorly (Figure 2–16 ■)
      4. Placed too far posteriorly (Figure 2–17 ■)

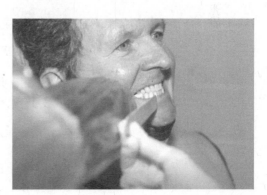

Figure 2–15 Using a tongue blade to visualize correct centering of the x-ray beam over the image receptor.

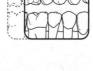

Figure 2–16 A horizontal molar bitewing radiograph demonstrating image receptor placed too far anteriorly so as not to record the distal contact between the second and third molars.

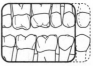

Figure 2–17 A horizontal premolar bitewing radiograph demonstrating image receptor placed too far posteriorly so as not to record the contact between the canines and the first premolars.

5. If not positioned (1) perpendicular to the embrasures and (2) parallel to the facial surfaces of the teeth of interest, incorrect horizontal angulation will result. (See horizontal angulation error described later in this section.)

B. Vertical angulation error
1. Occurs when the up-and-down angle of the PID is not set at +10 degrees when exposing bitewing radiographs on adults and +5 when exposing bitewing radiographs on children with primary dentition
2. Results in unequal distribution of the arches on the resultant radiograph
3. Excessive vertical angulation: angulation set greater than +10 degrees for adults and greater than +5 degrees for children (Figure 2–18 ■)
4. Inadequate vertical angulation: angulation set less than +10 degrees for adults and less than +5 degrees for children (Figure 2–19 ■)

C. Horizontal angulation error
1. Occurs when the side-to-side angulation of the PID is not set such that the x-ray beam will intersect with the image receptor perpendicularly through the embrasures of the teeth of interest; additionally, if the image receptor is not positioned (1) perpendicular to the embrasures and (2) parallel to the facial surfaces of the teeth of interest, the PID cannot be set such that the beam will intersect with the image receptor perpendicularly
2. Results in superimposition of proximal surfaces of adjacent teeth (overlap error)
3. Occurs when the x-ray beam intersects with the image receptor obliquely from the mesial direction (Figure 2–20 ■)
4. Occurs when the x-ray beam intersects with the image receptor obliquely from the distal direction (Figure 2–21 ■)

D. Centering the x-ray beam over the image receptor error
1. Occurs when the PID is not placed directly over the image receptor
2. Results in an unexposed or clear area recorded on the radiograph (conecut error)
3. Creates a conecut error when the beam is too far toward the anterior (Figure 2–22 ■)
4. Creates a conecut error when the beam is too far toward the posterior (Figure 2–23 ■)
5. Creates a conecut error when the beam is too far toward the superior (Figure 2–24 ■)
6. Creates a conecut error when the beam is too far toward the inferior (Figure 2–25 ■)

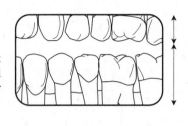

Figure 2–18 Excessive vertical angulation (greater than +10 degrees for an adult and greater than +5 degrees for a child with primary dentition) results in unequal distribution of the maxillary and mandibular arches, not recording the alveolar bone on the mandible.

Figure 2–19 Inadequate vertical angulation (less than +10 degrees for an adult and less than +5 degrees for a child with primary dentition) results in unequal distribution of the maxillary and mandibular arches, not recording the alveolar bone on the maxilla.

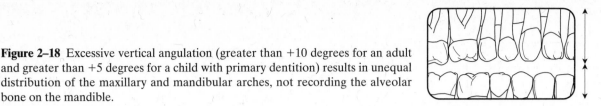

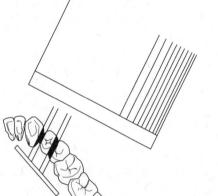

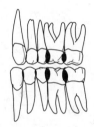

Figure 2–20 When the horizontal angulation intersects the image receptor obliquely from the mesial, the most severe overlap occurs in the posterior region of the image.

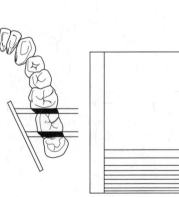

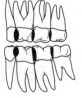

Figure 2–21 When the horizontal angulation intersects the image receptor obliquely from the distal, the most severe overlap occurs in the anterior region of the image.

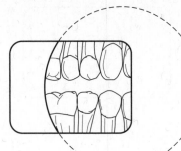

Figure 2–22 When the PID is not centered over the image receptor, an unexposed or clear "conecut" area results. When the conecut is in the posterior region of the image, the PID was positioned too far anteriorly.

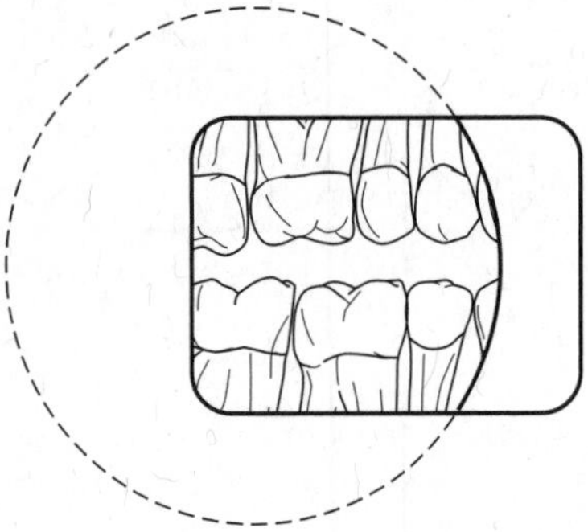

Figure 2–23 When the PID is not centered over the image receptor, an unexposed or clear "conecut" area results. When the conecut is in the anterior region of the image, the PID was positioned too far posteriorly.

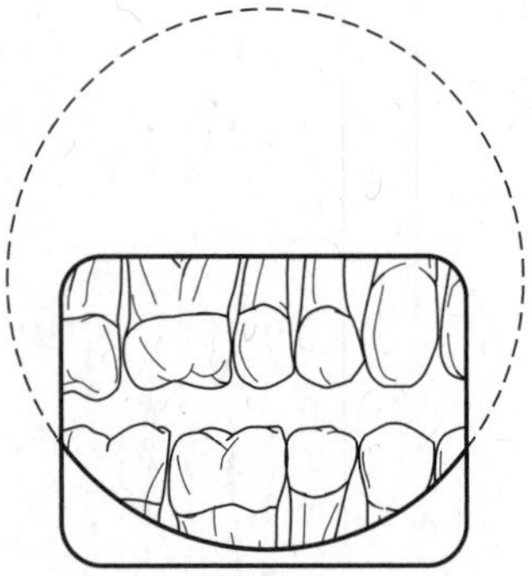

Figure 2–24 When the PID is not centered over the image receptor, an unexposed or clear "conecut" area results. When the conecut is in the inferior section of the image, the PID was positioned too far superiorly.

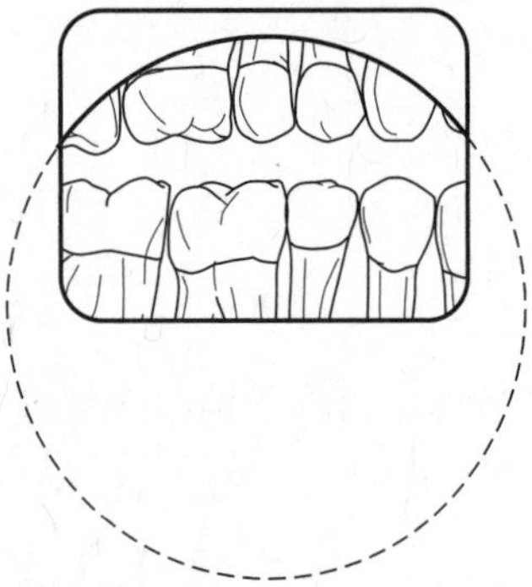

Figure 2–25 When the PID is not centered over the image receptor, an unexposed or clear "conecut" area results. When the conecut is in the superior section of the image, the PID was positioned too far inferiorly.

REFERENCES

Stabulas, J. J. (2002). Vertical bitewings: The other option. *Journal of Practical Hygiene,* 11, 46–47.

Thomson, E. M. (1993). Dental radiographs for the child patient. *Dental Hygienist News,* 6, 19–20, 24.

Thomson, E. M., & Johnson, O. N. (2012). *Essentials of dental radiography for dental assistants and hygienists* (9th ed.). Upper Saddle River, NJ: Pearson.

White, S. C., & Pharoah, M. J. (2008). *Oral radiology principles and interpretation* (6th ed.). St. Louis, MO: Elsevier.

1. Which of the following patients would benefit most from vertical bitewing radiographs rather than horizontal bitewing radiographs?
    A. Age 5 years, primary dentition, slight gingival inflammation, slight materia alba present
    B. Age 10 years, mixed dentition, moderate marginal and papillary gingivitis, moderate plaque present
    C. Age 25 years, permanent dentition, severe gingival inflammation, generalized probe readings of 5–8 mm
    D. Age 50 years, some missing teeth, generalized 1 mm recession, probing depths range from 1 mm to 2 mm

2. Which of the following teeth should be imaged on a horizontal premolar bitewing?
    A. Distal portion of the central incisor, lateral incisor, canine, first premolar, mesial portion of the second premolar
    B. Distal portion of the lateral incisor, canine, first premolar, second premolar, mesial portion of the first molar
    C. Distal portion of the canine, first premolar, second premolar, first molar, mesial portion of the second molar
    D. Distal portion of the first premolar, second premolar, first molar, second molar, mesial portion of the third molar

3. Which of the following teeth should be imaged on a horizontal molar bitewing?
    A. Distal portion of the lateral incisor, canine, first premolar, second premolar, mesial portion of the first premolar
    B. Distal portion of the canine, first premolar, second premolar, first molar, mesial portion of the second molar
    C. Distal portion of the first premolar, second premolar, first molar, second molar, mesial portion of the third molar
    D. Distal portion of the second premolar, first molar, second molar, third molar

4. With positive vertical angulation, the PID (position indicating device) is pointing such that the x-ray beam will be directed:
    A. Up
    B. Down

5. With negative vertical angulation, the PID (position indicating device) is pointing such that the x-ray beam will be directed:
    A. Up
    B. Down

6. Which of the following is the correct vertical angulation for bitewing radiographs on an adult patient?
    A. +10 degrees
    B. −10 degrees
    C. +15 degrees
    D. −15 degrees

7. Through which interproximal space should the central ray of the x-ray beam be directed when exposing a molar bitewing radiograph?
   A. Between the canine and the first premolar
   B. Between the first premolar and the second premolar
   C. Between the second premolar and the first molar
   D. Between the first molar and the second molar
   E. Between the second molar and the third molar

8. Overlapped interproximal spaces results from an error made in which of the following?
   A. Packet placement
   B. Vertical angulation
   C. Horizontal angulation
   D. Centering the x-ray beam

9. Unequal distribution of the arches (i.e., seeing more of the maxillary arch and not enough of the mandibular arch) results from an error made in which of the following?
   A. Packet placement
   B. Vertical angulation
   C. Horizontal angulation
   D. Centering the x-ray beam

10. Conecut error results from incorrect
    A. Packet placement
    B. Vertical angulation
    C. Horizontal angulation
    D. Centering the x-ray

laboratory exercise 3

Introduction to Digital Radiography

INTRODUCTION

One of today's technological advancements that is destined to improve the quality of oral health care is the use of digital radiography. Many practices have already made the transition from film-based radiography to digital imaging (Figure 3–1 ■). The radiology theories and imaging concepts for film-based radiography and digital imaging are basically the same. The difference between the two is the image receptor. Direct digital technology replaces film with a solid-state (meaning no moving parts) sensor made up of an electronic computer chip. Another type of indirect digital imaging technology called photostimuable phosphor or PSP replaces film with a plate covered with phosphor chemicals that capture the image and then release it as an electronic signal when stimulated by a laser light.

The purpose of this laboratory exercise is to introduce these two types of digital imaging technologies. While there are numerous digital imaging systems on the market, each will require the radiographer to be able to operate a computer, position the image receptor (sensor or phosphor plate) in the same manner as film, view radiographic images on a monitor, and utilize software to manipulate the images.

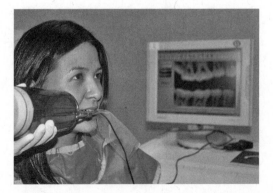

Figure 3–1 Radiographic procedure using digital imagery.

OBJECTIVES

Following completion of this lab activity, you will be able to:

1. Identify the components of a radiographic digital imaging system.

2. Place and expose a digital sensor and photostimuable phosphor (PSP) plate to produce a diagnostic quality image.

3. Maintain infection control during the radiographic procedure using a digital imaging system.

4. Demonstrate examples of digital image manipulation that will enhance the diagnostic quality of a digital radiograph.

MATERIALS

Teaching manikin or skull

Lead/lead equivalent apron with thyroid collar

Digital imaging system with one size #2 bitewing sensor

Indirect digital imaging system with four size #2 photostimuable phosphor (PSP) plates

Disinfectant and plastic barrier sheaths for the sensor and PSP plates (recommended by the manufacturer of the digital imaging system)

Bitewing image receptor holding device (recommended by the manufacturer of the digital imaging system)

Printer

PREPARATION

1. Study the chapter outline to prepare for this laboratory exercise. An understanding of the material presented in the outline is required to complete this activity.

2. Use Procedure 3–1 to assist you with completing the exercises. Your instructor may perform a demonstration to familiarize you with the digital system at your facility.

3. Prepare radiology operatory. Set up teaching manikin or skull. Ensure that correct "patient" positioning is achieved. Ensure that the occlusal plane is parallel to the floor and the midsagittal plane is perpendicular to the floor.

4. Place lead/lead equivalent barrier and thyroid collar over the "patient."

5. Obtain instructor feedback on your performance as necessary or as instructed.

LABORATORY EXERCISE ACTIVITIES

Part 1: Horizontal Bitewings Using Direct Digital Imaging

1. Turn on the computer. Using the keyboard or mouse, activate the exam window and select the template for four horizontal bitewing radiographs from the task bar.

2. Using the keyboard, type in the patient identification information with your name and your birthdate.

3. Prepare the sensor for placement intraorally.

4. Attach the sensor to the bitewing holder.

5. Check posted exposure settings for the dental x-ray machine and set for digital bitewing radiographs. See the manufacturer's recommendations for what settings to use with the digital system at your facility. Digital sensors currently available may require up to 50 percent less radiation than that required for F-speed film.

6. Place and expose the series of bitewing radiographs (see Table 2–1) in the following order:

1st	right premolar bitewing
2nd	right molar bitewing
3rd	left premolar bitewing
4th	left molar bitewing

   Note: Left-handed radiographers may use this order:

1st	left premolar bitewing
2nd	left molar bitewing
3rd	right premolar bitewing
4th	right molar bitewing

7. Observe the images on the computer monitor.

8. Remove the plastic barrier from the sensor and disinfect as recommended by the manufacturer.

Part 2: Horizontal Bitewings Using Indirect Digital Imaging

1. Turn on the computer. Using the keyboard or mouse, activate the exam window and select the template for four horizontal bitewing radiographs from the task bar.

2. Using the keyboard, type in the patient identification information with your name and your birthdate.

3. Prepare the PSP plates for placement intraorally.

4. Attach one of the PSP plates to the bitewing holder. The same holders that are used for film can usually be used to position PSP plates.

5. Check posted exposure settings for the dental x-ray machine and set for digital bitewing radiographs. See the manufacturer's recommendations for what settings to use with the digital system at your facility. PSP plates have a wide latitude of acceptable exposure, meaning that the computer will self-adjust the image if under- or overexposed. Carefully choose the lowest setting possible to avoid unnecessary excess radiation exposure. PSP plates may require slightly higher exposure settings than direct digital sensors to avoid the appearance of radiographic noise, a condition similar to film fog.

6. Place and expose the series of bitewing radiographs (see Table 2–1) in the following order:

   1st   right premolar bitewing

   2nd   right molar bitewing

   3rd   left premolar bitewing

   4th   left molar bitewing

   Note: Left-handed radiographers may use this order:

   1st   left premolar bitewing

   2nd   left molar bitewing

   3rd   right premolar bitewing

   4th   right molar bitewing

7. Remove the plastic barrier envelopes from the PSP plates and disinfect as recommended by the manufacturer.

8. Place the PSP plates in the containment box or face down on the counter to protect from bright light until the four exposures are complete.

9. Place all four PSP plates into the laser scanner (see Figure 1–8).

10. Observe the images on the computer monitor.

11. If the scanning process did not automatically erase the PSP plates, expose the used plates to a bright light source such as a view box to erase.

Part 3: Interpretation of Digital Images

1. Evaluate the images obtained in Parts 1 and 2.

2. Print one hard copy each of the bitewing radiographic exams obtained with both direct and indirect digital imaging. Do not close the file.

3. Next, experiment with using the computer software to change the following on each of the sets of bitewing radiographs:
   a. Right molar bitewing—increase the density
   b. Right premolar bitewing—increase the contrast
   c. Left premolar bitewing—enlarge the image (magnification tool)

    d. Left molar bitewing—manipulate the image using one of the software tools such as reversing the gray scale, embossing, colorization, and so on.

4. Print one hard copy of the manipulated bitewing radiographic images.

COMPETENCY AND EVALUATION

1. Obtain instructor feedback. Identify which step (packet placement, vertical angulation, horizontal angulation, centering) needs improvement.

2. Repeat Part 1 and Part 2 at the direction of your instructor.

3. Examine the first printout of your digital images. Evaluate your technique. Are the radiographic images diagnostic? Were you able to transfer the skills you learned with film-based radiography to this technology? What did you discover to be the most challenging aspect of digital radiographic technology? What is your opinion of this technology? Do you prefer one, direct digital imaging, indirect digital imaging, or film-based radiography, over the other? Why? Which do you think patients will prefer? What advantages and disadvantages did you encounter using this technology for this exercise?

4. Examine the second printout of your digital images. What are the advantages and disadvantages of the software tools utilized for this exercise? Did the system mark the second printout as a manipulated image? What might be the legal ramifications of digital imagery?

5. Complete the study questions.

Procedure 3–1

Digital Radiographic Procedure

1. Activate computer exam window.
   a. Turn on the computer.
   b. Open the digital imaging system program from the desktop window.
   c. Choose "new exam" from the task bar.
   d. Type your name (*last and first*) into the patient name box. If required, type your birthdate as the patient identification number.
   e. Choose the four horizontal bitewings template.
2. Prepare sensor or PSP plate for placement intraorally.
   a. Wipe with an appropriate intermediate-level disinfectant recommended by the manufacturer. Place a plastic barrier sheath (for wired sensors) (Figure 3–2 ■) or plastic barrier envelop (for wireless sensors and for phosphor plates) (Figure 3–3 ■) that is recommended by the manufacturer over the image receptor.
   b. Choose the appropriate image receptor holder recommended by the manufacturer and attach to the image receptor (Figure 3–4 ■ and 3–5 ■).
3. Turn on the x-ray machine and adjust the exposure settings.
   a. See the manufacturer's recommendation. Exposure time may possibly be reduced up to one-half the exposure time required for F-speed film.
4. Place the image receptor into position intraorally.

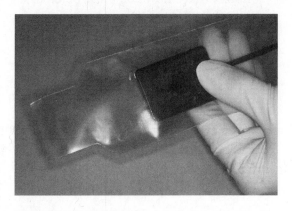

Figure 3–2 Wired digital sensor being covered with a plastic barrier sheath.

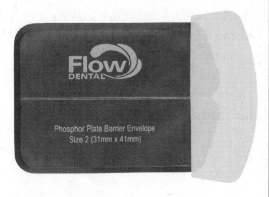

Figure 3–3 Plastic barrier envelope for a photostimuable phosphor (PSP) plate.

(continued)

Procedure 3–1 (continued)

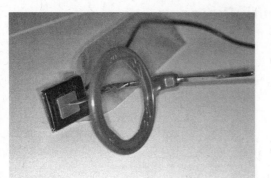

Figure 3–4 A wired sensor attached to a holder, ready for positioning intraorally.

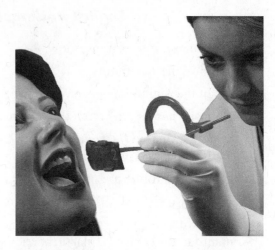

Figure 3–5 Phosphor plate attached to a holder, ready for positioning intraorally. (Courtesy of Gendex Dental Systems)

Direct digital sensor technology

5. Highlight the box representing the first exposure. (Figure 3–6 ■) Ensure that you place the sensor into the position that is highlighted on the template. If not, you will have to drag-and-drop the image into the correct space on the template later.

6. Activate the exposure button.

7. Wait for the image to appear on the computer monitor and evaluate. Do not remove the sensor from the patient's mouth yet.

Indirect digital phosphor plate technology

5. Activate the exposure button.

6. Remove the PSP plate from the oral cavity.

7. Remove the PSP plate from the holding device and place into a containment box or face down on the protected work surface to avoid exposure to bright ambient room lighting.

8. Repeat steps 4 through 7 with the other three PSP plates to expose the set of four horizontal bitewing radiographs.

(continued)

Procedure 3-1 (continued)

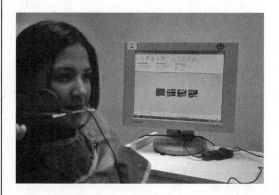

Figure 3–6 Highlighted box indicating that the next exposure will be the right molar bitewing radiograph.

8. If a technique error has occurred and a retake is required, adjust the sensor position or the PID angle to correct the error noted without completely removing the sensor from the patient's mouth.

9. Follow the digital software program instructions to retake the image and activate the re-exposure. Repeat steps 6 through 8 to produce a diagnostic quality image.

10. When the images are satisfactory, reposition the sensor for the next exposure and repeat steps 4 through 8 until all four bitewing radiographs have been exposed.

11. Remove the sensor from the holding device. Remove the sensor from the plastic barrier sheath and clean and disinfect according to the manufacturer's instructions

12. Save the bitewing radiographic examination in the archived files. Back up the file on a supplemental storage system.

9. Remove the PSP plates from the plastic barrier envelopes and clean and disinfect according to the manufacturer's instructions.

10. Keep the four PSP plates in a containment box until ready for scanning (Figure 3–7 ■) or place directly into the laser scanner and activate (see Figure 1–8). Follow manufacturer's instructions for the order and orientation of the plates in placing them into the scanner so that the images will be positioned appropriately into the template on the computer monitor. This will avoid having to drag-and-drop the images to the correct position later.

11. Observe the images on the computer monitor and evaluate technique. If a technique error has occurred and a retake is required be sure that the PSP plate has been erased prior to using it again.

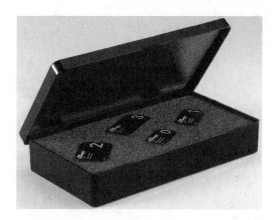

Figure 3–7 Containment box holding exposed phosphor plates until ready for scanning. (Courtesy of Air Techniques, Inc.)

I. Digital radiographic imaging technology
   A. Digital versus analog (Figure 3–8 ■)
      1. Black-and-white film-based radiographs are considered analog because the distribution of the silver halide crystals create a continuous density pattern.
      2. Digital refers to a numeric format of the image; distinct pixels (*pix,* plural of *pic*ture and *el,* short for *el*ement) create the image.
      3. Digital images have no physical form but exist as numerical data in a computer file.
   B. Fundamentals (Figure 3–1)
      1. Film is replaced with an electronic sensor or phosphor-coated silicon chip. Sensors and photostimuable phosphor (PSP) plates are available in sizes that approximate film sizes.
      2. An electronic charge is produced on the surface of the image receptor that is digitized and transmitted to a computer.
      3. The computer processes the signal and produces an image on a monitor.
      4. While dental x-ray machines with low milliamperage and low kilovoltage settings of 5 mA and 70 kVp or less are ideal for use with digital imaging, all conventional dental x-ray machines may be used for both film-based and digital radiography.
   C. Methods of acquiring a digital image
      1. Direct digital imaging
         a. This technology uses an image receptor called a solid-state (meaning no moving parts) sensor containing an electronic chip.
            1) Charge-coupled device (CCD) technology
            2) Complementary metal oxide semiconductor (CMOS) technology
            3) Both CCD and CMOS technologies work equally well at converting x-rays into an electronic signal. The use of CCD or CMOS technology depends on the manufacturer of the digital imaging system.
         b. Pixels arranged in a matrix (the pixels are the silver halide equivalent of film) on a silicon surface act as "wells" into which radiation is deposited creating the latent image.

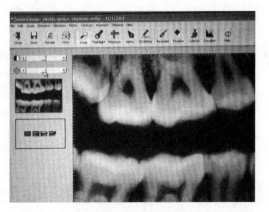

Figure 3–8 Example of a digital radiographic image. Note the computer software task bar and icons that allow the operator to adjust and manipulate the image.

     c. The latent image is then transferred to the computer via a wire or wirelessly via radio frequency.

     d. The computer reconstructs the numerical data captured by the pixels into a visible radiographic image on the monitor.

  2. Indirect digital imaging

     a. This technology is called photostimuable phosphor (PSP) technology.

     b. It uses a phosphor-coated plate as the image receptor that absorbs and stores x-ray energy until later released as light (phosphorescence) when stimulated with a laser scanner device.

     c. Phosphor plates "store" the x-ray energy similar to the way silver halide crystals within film emulsion store a latent image.

     d. The laser scanning step required for PSP technology is often compared to the processing step required for film-based imaging.

     e. The laser scanner, connected to a computer, "processes" the data by sending an electronic signal from the released light to a computer.

     f. The computer reconstructs the numerical data in the electronic signal into a visible radiographic image on the monitor.

     g. Phosphor plates must be erased by exposing them to a bright light source prior to reusing. The laser scanner may have a setting that conveniently automatically erases the plates after sending the signal to the computer. If no setting is available, the plates may be erased by placing them, front side down, on a bright light source such as a viewbox.

D. Computer

  1. This is responsible for converting the numerical data into an image that can be viewed on a monitor; it should provide adequate storage

  2. Images are available for viewing on the computer monitor within 0.5 to 120 seconds following exposure.

  3. All monitor types (large, older cathode ray tube [CRT] monitors, with tested technology and newer flat-panel monitors, including plasma and liquid crystal display [LCD] screens) are all considered acceptable for viewing digital radiographic images.

  4. An Internet connection allows for electronic transfer of images between practices for consultations and referrals or to third-party payment providers for approval of treatment.

E. Software

  1. Images may be viewed side-by-side, compared with images obtained previously, and enlarged or magnified.

  2. The ability to manipulate images for the purpose of enhancing diagnosis includes adjusting the density or contrast, measurement tools for endodontic procedures and determining periodontal bone loss, charting and notations for treatment planning and documentation, and digital subtraction:

     a. This is a process by which two images acquired at different points in treatment may be superimposed on each other.

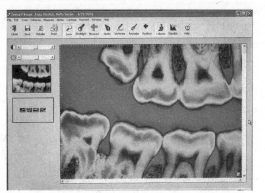

Figure 3–9 Software used to manipulate the image.

        b. Unchanged anatomy will cancel out of the image, leaving changes to appear distinctly.

        c. It is valuable in assessing periodontal bone loss or regeneration.

        d. Technological advances in software that match gray values between subsequent images have made digital subtraction easier to achieve.

    3. Other software features include reversing the gray scale, embossing, and colorization. Some practitioners find that changing the way the image appears on the screen aids in diagnosis, although this is not currently supported by research (Figure 3–9 ■).

    4. Software programs may imprint manipulated images with an identification that labels the image as changed from the original.

II. Characteristics of a digital image

  A. Contrast

    1. This allows the viewer to distinguish between different densities (light or dark areas) on the image.

    2. Dental digital sensors are capable of capturing 256 to over 65,000 different densities.

    3. Computer monitors reserve the use of some gray levels for their operating system, so most computer monitors currently available only display about 242 levels of gray.

    4. The human eye is capable of detecting about 30 levels of gray.

    5. Due to its ability to record many levels of gray, there is potential for the computer to aid in diagnosis. However, current software programs are not able to do this better than the human practitioner.

  B. Spatial resolution

    1. This is defined as the ability to distinguish between closely spaced objects.

    2. The number and size of the pixels determines spatial resolution.

    3. Fewer pixels produce an image with jagged edges. More pixels produce a smoother image.

    4. Spatial resolution is measured in line pairs per millimeter (lp/mm).

        a. It is defined as the ability to distinguish between very fine sets of radiopaque lines.

        b. The greater the spatial resolution, the sharper the image.

        c. The unaided human eye can distinguish between approximately 60 lp/mm.

        d. Film-based radiographs record approximately 200 lp/mm.

        e. Digital images displayed on a computer monitor reveal approximately 70 lp/mm.

        f. When software is utilized to magnify a digital image, the image begins to look jagged and take on a "building block" appearance, indicating the limited spatial resolution obtained with digital radiography.

III. Advantages and limitations of digital imaging compared with film-based radiography

  A. Advantages

    1. Digital sensors are more sensitive to radiation than film, requiring between 0 to 50 percent less radiation dose to the patient when compared to fast-speed film. However, currently there is no rating system to classify the speed of digital image receptors so these reductions in radiation exposure are based on limited research and often on manufacturers' claims.

    2. Instant viewing of the image saves time and aids in correcting errors when retakes are necessary.

    3. Digital imaging eliminates the need for darkroom, chemicals, and the generation of lead foil and silver halide wastes.

    4. It has the potential to improve the image without re-exposing the patient (density and contrast may be improved through the use of software).

    5. Improved gray scale has the potential to aid in diagnosis.

    6. Electronic transfer of images via the Internet speeds communication between professionals and third-party payment providers.

    7. It can enhance patient education, using the computer monitor to view the images.

  B. Limitations

    1. There is the potential for increased radiation exposure. The real and perceived reduction in radiation exposure coupled with an instant view of the images is purported to make retakes seem easily justifiable.

    2. Smaller recording size of the image receptor may present a need for additional exposures. Larger physical dimensions of wired and wireless sensors and the need for sheathing the sensor within an infection control barrier may interfere with precise positioning intraorally on some patients.

    3. Unless the practitioner learned digital imaging in his or her professional educational setting, a learning curve is required to transfer technique and interpretative skills from film-based radiography to digital imaging.

    4. The practice can incur investment costs if converting from a film-based practice. However, when starting a new practice, the costs of setting up with digital imaging (with its savings in not having to purchase film and processing chemicals or dispose of hazardous wastes) may be comparable to setting up a film-based practice.

    5. The issue of timing when to purchase the system is important. As technology advances, equipment may become dated or obsolete in a relatively short time.

6. The issue of reliability of computer-stored patient records is also important. The possibility of record loss due to computer crashes, system malfunction, and computer viruses is a real risk.
7. Although environmentally friendly in the short term, disposal of broken, obsolete digital equipment is a concern.

IV. Digital Imaging and Communications in Medicine (DICOM)
   A. This is the standard to allow different digital systems to interface with each other.
   B. Exporting and importing digital images can require complex steps and considerable computer knowledge. Without standards, system compatibility would be an issue when digital images are transferred electronically between systems.
   C. Currently manufacturers of dental digital imaging systems are being encouraged to produce systems that are compatible with each other.

REFERENCES

American Dental Association Standards Committee on Dental Informatics. (2005). *Implementation requirements for DICOM in dentistry.* Technical report no. 1023-2005.

Farman, A. G., & Farman, T. T. (2005). A comparison of 18 different x-ray detectors currently used in dentistry. *Oral Surg, Oral Med, Oral Path,* 99, 485–489.

Francisco, E. F., Horlak, D., & Azevedo, S. (2010). The balance between safety and efficacy: Understanding the technology available that will produce high quality radiographs while reducing patient risk to ionizing radiation. *Dimen Dent Hyg,* 8, 26–30.

Horner, K., Drage, N., & Brettle, D. (2008). *21st century imaging.* London: Quintessence Publishing Co., Ltd.

Palenik, C. J. (2004). Infection control for dental radiography. *Dentistry Today,* 23, 52–55.

Thomson, E. M., & Johnson, O. N. (2012). *Essentials of dental radiography for dental assistants and hygienists* (9th ed.). Upper Saddle River, NJ: Pearson.

Van der Stelt, P. F. (2008). Better imaging: the advantages of digital radiography. *J Am Dent Assoc,* 139, 7S–13S.

White, S. C., & Pharoah, M. J. (2008). *Oral radiology principles and interpretation* (6th ed.). St. Louis, MO: Elsevier.

Williamson, G. F. (2005). Digital radiography in dentistry. *J Pract Hyg,* 13–14.

STUDY QUESTIONS

1. Distinct pixels, arranged numerically to form a radiographic image, are referred to as a (an)
   - A. Analog image.
   - B. Digital image.
   - C. Latent image.
   - D. Film-based image.

2. A _____ is used to capture x-radiation as an electronic charge that a computer will convert to a radiographic image for viewing on a monitor.
   - A. Software program
   - B. Radio frequency
   - C. Scanner
   - D. Sensor

3. Which of the following is considered ideal for producing digital radiographic images?
   - A. 70 kVp, 5 mA
   - B. 70 kVp, 15 mA
   - C. 90 kVp, 5 mA
   - D. 90 kVp, 15 mA

4. Which of the following types of image receptors requires a "processing" step where the image receptor must be read using a laser scanner?
   - A. CCD
   - B. CMOS
   - C. PSP

5. Each of the following must be performed on a photostimuable phosphor (PSP) plate image receptor prior to reusing it to expose a radiograph EXCEPT one. Which one is the EXCEPTION?
   - A. Calibrate it with the computer software.
   - B. Wipe it with an intermediate-level disinfectant.
   - C. Place it in a plastic barrier envelope.
   - D. Expose it to bright light to erase the data.

6. The human eye can detect about 242 levels of gray.
   A digital image displayed on a computer monitor may contain up to 30 levels of gray.
   - A. The first statement is true. The second statement is false.
   - B. The first statement is false. The second statement is true.
   - C. Both statements are true.
   - D. Both statements are false.

7. Which of the following terms is defined as the ability to distinguish between closely spaced objects?
   - A. Contrast
   - B. Density
   - C. Spatial resolution
   - D. Sensitivity
   - E. Gray level

8. Each of the following is true EXCEPT one. Which one is the EXCEPTION?

   A. The unaided human eye can detect approximately 60 lp/mm.
   B. A phosphor plate can capture approximately 500 lp/mm.
   C. A computer monitor can display approximately 70 lp/mm.
   D. Film-based radiography can record approximately 200 lp/mm.

9. Each of the following is considered an advantage of digital imaging when compared with film-based imaging EXCEPT one. Which one is the EXCEPTION?

   A. Less radiation required.
   B. Less time required to produce an image.
   C. Digital sensor size records a larger area.
   D. Electronic transfer of images facilitates consultations.
   E. Image contrast and density can be improved without reexposing the patient.

10. Each of the following is considered a limitation of digital imaging when compared with film-based imaging EXCEPT one. Which one is the EXCEPTION?

   A. Learning curve to transfer technique and interpretative skills from film-based radiography.
   B. Physical size of the sensor may interfere with positioning on some patients.
   C. Computer malfunction can produce catastrophic record loss.
   D. The ease of retakes may result in excess radiation exposure.
   E. Images contain more gray shade levels.

Periapical Radiographs— Paralleling Technique

INTRODUCTION

A dental radiographic examination plays an important role in identifying and diagnosing oral conditions. Periapical radiographs are particularly useful in that they image the entire tooth from incisal/occlusal edge to the tip of the tooth root. There are two radiographic techniques used to expose periapical radiographs, and the dental radiographer should develop skills necessary for both. The technique recommended by the American Dental Association and the American Academy of Oral and Maxillofacial Radiology for exposing periapical radiographs is the paralleling technique. Periapical radiographs taken utilizing the paralleling technique are more likely to be free of the image distortion typically found with the bisecting technique.

The same four basic steps—packet placement, vertical angulation, horizontal angulation, and centering the x-ray beam—that are utilized when placing and exposing bitewing radiographs (Laboratory Exercise 2, Bitewing Radiographic Technique) are employed when placing and exposing periapical radiographs. Learning the paralleling technique by following these four distinct steps will help the radiographer consistently produce diagnostic quality periapical radiographs. Additionally, evaluation of the radiographic image is easier when errors can be attributed to a specific step. Identification of which step is the cause of an error will help pinpoint which skill needs concentrated practice efforts. The simulated mount pages provided in this laboratory exercise may be copied to increase the amount of practice sessions required to master the techniques.

There are a variety of commercially made film and digital sensor holding devices on the market. This beginning exercise uses a disposable, polystyrene biteblock film holder, Stabe® (Dentsply Rinn) (Figure 4–1 ■) for film-based radiography. The use of this holder requires a working knowledge of appropriate angles. Mastering these skills with an understanding of projection geometry will allow you to easily transfer this working knowledge to other periapical image receptor holding devices such as the one noted in Figure 4–2 ■. Commercially available image receptor holding devices designed with external aiming devices are valuable aids to determining

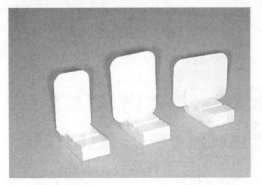

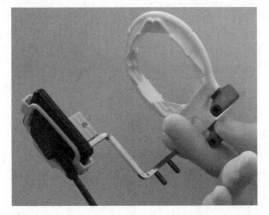

Figure 4–1 Stabe® disposable polystyrene film holder with size #1 and size #2 films placed vertically for anterior periapical radiographs and placed horizontally for posterior periapical radiographs.

Figure 4–2 Periapical radiographic image receptor holder with external aiming device. Note the use of a digital image receptor.

appropriate angles and points of entry. However, the bulk and weight of the attachments may make the device difficult to position precisely on some patients. This may be true for children, adults with small or sensitive oral cavities or intrusive tori, or the patient with a hypersensitive gag reflex. If these image receptor holders are positioned incorrectly, the x-ray beam will be aligned inaccurately. The radiographer who can recognize accurate beam alignment without the use of an external aiming device may be better able to evaluate the position of any image receptor holder, regardless of type.

OBJECTIVES

Following completion of this lab activity, you will be able to:

1. Demonstrate proficiency in placing, exposing, and processing anterior and posterior periapical radiographs using the paralleling technique.

2. Critique a full mouth series of intraoral radiographs consisting of anterior and posterior periapicals for correct (a) placement of the image receptor intraorally, (b) vertical and (c) horizontal angulation of the PID, and (d) direction of the x-ray beam over the entire image receptor.

MATERIALS

Teaching manikin or skull

Lead/lead equivalent apron with thyroid collar

Size #1 and size #2 radiographic films (or digital image receptors)

Periapical film holding device (disposable Stabe® or similar device designed for use with the paralleling technique)

Viewbox

Tongue blades

PREPARATION

1. Study the chapter outline to prepare for this laboratory exercise. An understanding of the material presented in the outline is required to complete this activity.

2. Use Table 4–1 to assist you in completing the exercises. Instructor demonstration may enhance knowledge of the laboratory exercise.

3. Prepare radiology operatory. Set up teaching manikin or skull. Ensure that correct "patient" positioning is achieved. To image the maxilla, ensure that the maxillary occlusal plane is parallel to the floor; to image the mandible, ensure that the mandibular occlusal plane is parallel to the floor and the midsagittal plane must be perpendicular to the floor for both maxillary and mandibular exposures.

4. Place lead/lead equivalent barrier and thyroid collar over the "patient."

5. The size and/or number of image receptors included in a full mouth series of periapical radiographs varies among practices. The anterior periapical radiographic examination may include the exposure of six, seven, or eight periapical radiographs, whereas the posterior radiographic examination usually remains standard with the exposure of eight periapical radiographs (Figure 4–3 ■). This exercise will focus on the use of two of the most common full mouth series configurations: Figures 4–3A and 4–3B.

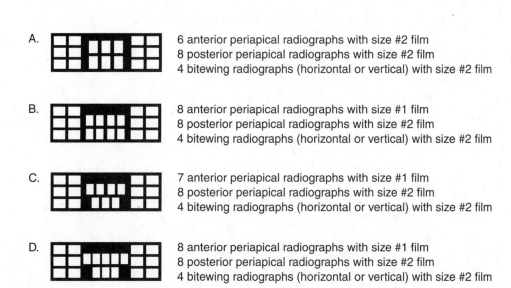

A. 6 anterior periapical radiographs with size #2 film
8 posterior periapical radiographs with size #2 film
4 bitewing radiographs (horizontal or vertical) with size #2 film

B. 8 anterior periapical radiographs with size #1 film
8 posterior periapical radiographs with size #2 film
4 bitewing radiographs (horizontal or vertical) with size #2 film

C. 7 anterior periapical radiographs with size #1 film
8 posterior periapical radiographs with size #2 film
4 bitewing radiographs (horizontal or vertical) with size #2 film

D. 8 anterior periapical radiographs with size #1 film
8 posterior periapical radiographs with size #2 film
4 bitewing radiographs (horizontal or vertical) with size #2 film

Figure 4–3 Four examples of full mouth series.

TABLE 4–1 Summary of Steps for Acquiring Periapical Radiographs for Adult Patients—Paralleling Technique

Periapical Radiograph	Packet Placement	Vertical Angulation	Horizontal Angulation	Centering
Maxillary Central-Lateral Incisors (Figure 4–3, series configuration A) Use image receptor size #1 or size #2	Center the image receptor to line up behind the central and lateral incisors on both the right and left sides; if using a size #2 image receptor, include the mesial halves of the canines (Figure 4–4 ■).	Direct the central rays of the x-ray beam toward the image receptor perpendicularly in the vertical dimension; the PID will be pointing down.	Direct the central rays of the x-ray beam perpendicularly through the left and right central incisor embrasure (Figure 4–5 ■).	Center the image receptor within the x-ray beam; direct the central rays of the x-ray beam toward the center of the image receptor.
Maxillary Central-Lateral Incisors (Figure 4–3, series configuration B) Use image receptor size #1	Center the image receptor to line up behind the central and lateral incisors on one side of the mouth; include a portion of the central incisor on the opposite side and a portion of the canine (Figure 4–6 ■).	Direct the central rays of the x-ray beam toward the image receptor perpendicularly in the vertical dimension; the PID will be pointing down.	Direct the central rays of the x-ray beam perpendicularly through the central incisor and lateral incisor embrasure (Figure 4–5).	Center the image receptor within the x-ray beam; direct the central rays of the x-ray beam toward the center of the image receptor.
Maxillary Canine (Figure 4–3, same for both series configurations A & B) Use image receptor size #1 or size #2	Center the image receptor to line up behind the canine; include the distal half of the lateral incisor and the mesial half of the first premolar (Figures 4–4 and 4–6).	Direct the central rays of the x-ray beam toward the image receptor perpendicularly in the vertical dimension; the PID will be pointing down.	Direct the central rays of the x-ray beam perpendicularly in the horizontal direction at the center of the canine (Figure 4–5).	Center the image receptor within the x-ray beam; direct the central rays of the x-ray beam toward the center of the image receptor.
Maxillary Premolar (Figure 4–3, same for both series configurations A & B) Use image receptor size #2	Align the anterior edge of image receptor to line up behind the distal half of the canine; include the first and second premolars, first molar, and mesial half of the second molar (Figure 4–7 ■).	Direct the central rays of the x-ray beam toward the image receptor perpendicularly in the vertical dimension; the PID will be pointing down.	Direct the central rays of the x-ray beam perpendicularly through the first and second premolar embrasure (Figure 4–5).	Center the image receptor within the x-ray beam; direct the central rays of the x-ray beam toward the center of the image receptor.
Maxillary Molar (Figure 4–3, same for both series configurations A & B) Use image receptor size #2	Align the anterior edge of image receptor to line up behind the distal half of the second premolar; include the first, second, and third molars (Figure 4–7).	Direct the central rays of the x-ray beam toward the image receptor perpendicularly in the vertical dimension; the PID will be pointing down.	Direct the central rays of the x-ray beam perpendicularly through the first and second molar embrasure (Figure 4–5).	Center the image receptor within the x-ray beam; direct the central rays of the x-ray beam toward the center of the image receptor.

Tooth	Image Receptor Placement	Vertical Angulation	Horizontal Angulation	Centering
Mandibular Central-Lateral Incisors (Figure 4–3, series configuration A) Use image receptor size #1 or size #2	Center the image receptor to line up behind the central and lateral incisors; if using a size #2 image receptor, include the mesial halves of the canines (Figure 4–4).	Direct the central rays of the x-ray beam toward the image receptor perpendicularly in the vertical dimension; the PID will be pointing up.	Direct the central rays of the x-ray beam perpendicularly through the left and right central incisor embrasure (Figure 4–5).	Center the image receptor within the x-ray beam; direct the central rays of the x-ray beam toward the center of the image receptor.
Mandibular Central-Lateral Incisors (Figure 4–3, series configuration B) Use image receptor size #1	Center the image receptor to line up behind the central and lateral incisors on one side of the mouth; include a portion of the central incisor on the opposite side and a portion of the canine (Figure 4–6).	Direct the central rays of the x-ray beam toward the image receptor perpendicularly in the vertical dimension; the PID will be pointing up.	Direct the central rays of the x-ray beam perpendicularly through the central incisor and lateral incisor embrasure (Figure 4–5).	Center the image receptor within the x-ray beam; direct the central rays of the x-ray beam toward the center of the image receptor.
Mandibular Canine (Figure 4–3, same for both series configurations A & B) Use image receptor size #1 or size #2	Center the image receptor to line up behind the canine; include the distal half of the lateral incisor and the mesial half of the first premolar (Figures 4–4 and 4–6).	Direct the central rays of the x-ray beam toward the image receptor perpendicularly in the vertical dimension; the PID will be pointing up.	Direct the central rays of the x-ray beam perpendicularly in the horizontal direction at the center of the canine (Figure 4–5).	Center the image receptor within the x-ray beam; direct the central rays of the x-ray beam toward the center of the image receptor.
Mandibular Premolar (Figure 4–3, same for both series configurations A & B) Use image receptor size #2	Align the anterior edge of image receptor to line up behind the distal half of the canine; include the first and second premolars and mesial half of the first molar (Figure 4–7).	Direct the central rays of the x-ray beam toward the image receptor perpendicularly in the vertical dimension; the PID will be pointing up.	Direct the central rays of the x-ray beam perpendicularly through the first and second premolar embrasure (Figure 4–5).	Center the image receptor within the x-ray beam; direct the central rays of the x-ray beam toward the center of the image receptor.
Mandibular Molar (Figure 4–3, same for both series configurations A & B) Use image receptor size #2	Align the anterior edge of image receptor to line up behind the distal half of the second premolar; include the first, second, and third molars (Figure 4–7).	Direct the central rays of the x-ray beam toward the image receptor perpendicularly in the vertical dimension; the PID will be pointing up.	Direct the central rays of the x-ray beam perpendicularly through the first and second molar embrasure (Figure 4–5).	Center the image receptor within the x-ray beam; direct the central rays of the x-ray beam toward the center of the image receptor.

Source: Thomson, E. M., & Johnson, O. N. (2012). *Essentials of dental radiography for dental assistants and hygienists* (9th ed.). Upper Saddle River, NJ: Pearson.

Maxillary Central-Lateral Incisors

Maxillary Canine

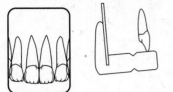 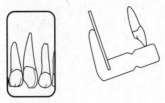

Mandibular Central-Lateral Incisors

Mandibular Canine

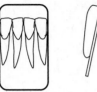 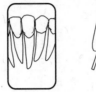

Figure 4–4 Full mouth series A—image receptor placements for anterior periapical radiographs.

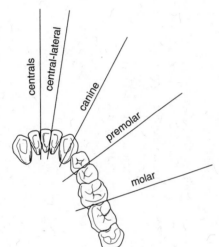

Figure 4–5 Horizontal angulation for central incisors, central-lateral incisors, canine, premolar, and molar periapical radiographs can be determined by directing the central ray of the x-ray beam perpendicularly between a predetermined interproximal space.

Maxillary Central-Lateral Incisors

Maxillary Canine

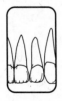   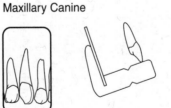

Mandibular Central-Lateral Incisors

Mandibular Canine

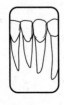

Figure 4–6 Full mouth series B—image receptor placements for anterior periapical radiographs.

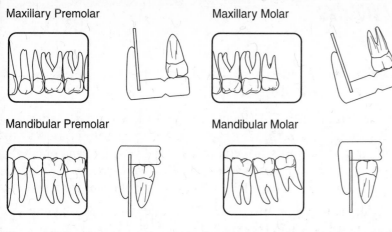

Maxillary Premolar

Maxillary Molar

Mandibular Premolar

Mandibular Molar

Figure 4–7 Image receptor placements for posterior periapical radiographs. Note that the bite extension of the holder may be shortened in the **mandibular posterior** region *only*. The very nearly straight position or slight lingual tilt of the posterior teeth (molars and premolars) within the mandibular arch allows a close relationship between the lingual surfaces of the teeth and the image receptor to remain parallel. In the mandibular anterior region and both anterior and posterior regions of the maxillary, the biteblock extension is necessary for parallel relationship between teeth and plane of the image receptor.

6. Obtain disposable Stabe® periapical film holders or similar device designed for use with the paralleling technique.

7. If using film, orient into the holder so that the embossed identification dot will be placed away from the apices of the teeth. Place the "dot in the slot" of the film holder to position the identification dot of the film packet toward the incisal/occlusal edges of the teeth (Figure 4–8 ■). If using photostimuable phosphor (PSP) plates or digital sensor, orient so that the appropriate side faces the x-ray beam.

8. Start with the anterior exposures. Beginning the examination with the more tolerable anterior placements will help to gain the patient's confidence and cooperation with the procedure.

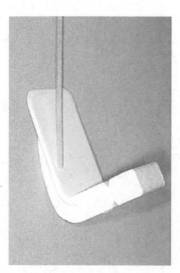

Figure 4–8 Place the embossed identification dot into the film retention groove of the film holder when placing a periapical film packet intraorally to keep it away from the area of interest, which is the root apices.

LABORATORY EXERCISE ACTIVITIES

Part 1: Periapical Radiographs Using the Paralleling Technique—Anterior Region

1. If using *Full Mouth Series A* (Figure 4–3A) for this exercise, you may choose to obtain six size #2 radiographic image receptors, six size #1 radiographic image receptors, or a combination of five size #1 and one size #2 radiographic image receptors. If using *Full Mouth Series B* (Figure 4–3B) for this exercise, obtain eight size #1 radiographic image receptors.

2. Place the image receptor into the Stabe® holder with the long dimension positioned vertically. (Figure 4–1)

3. Check posted exposure settings for the dental x-ray machine prior to placing each image receptor and set for the anterior region; adjust as needed for the maxilla, for the mandible, and for the canine and the central incisor regions.

4. Place and expose the anterior periapical radiographs in the following order:

Full Mouth Series A (Figure 4–3A)

1st	right maxillary canine
2nd	maxillary central incisors
3rd	left maxillary canine
4th	left mandibular canine
5th	mandibular central incisors
6th	right mandibular canine

Full Mouth Series B (Figure 4–3B)

1st	right maxillary canine
2nd	right maxillary central-lateral incisors
3rd	left maxillary central-lateral incisors
4th	left maxillary canine
5th	left mandibular canine
6th	left mandibular central-lateral incisors
7th	right mandibular central-lateral incisors
8th	right mandibular canine

Note: Left-handed radiographers may use this order:

Full Mouth Series A (Figure 4–3A)

1st	left maxillary canine
2nd	maxillary central incisors
3rd	right maxillary canine
4th	right mandibular canine

| 5th | mandibular central incisors |
| 6th | left mandibular canine |

Full Mouth Series B (Figure 4–3B)

1st	left maxillary canine
2nd	left maxillary central-lateral incisors
3rd	right maxillary central-lateral incisors
4th	right maxillary canine
5th	right mandibular canine
6th	right mandibular central-lateral incisors
7th	left mandibular central-lateral incisors
8th	left mandibular canine

5. Process the films or scan the PSP plates or observe the digital images on computer monitor.

Part 2: Periapical Radiographs Using the Paralleling Technique—Posterior Region

1. Obtain eight size #2 image receptors. All full mouth series configurations on adult patients will most likely use the same standard eight posterior image receptor placements.

2. Place image receptor into the Stabe® holder with the long dimension positioned horizontally (Figure 4–1).

3. Check posted exposure settings for the dental x-ray machine prior to placing each image receptor and set for the posterior region; adjust as needed for the maxilla, for the mandible, and for the premolar and molar regions.

4. Place and expose the posterior periapical radiographs in the following order:

1st	right maxillary premolar
2nd	right maxillary molar
3rd	right mandibular premolar
4th	right mandibular molar
5th	left maxillary premolar
6th	left maxillary molar
7th	left mandibular premolar
8th	left mandibular molar

Note: Left-handed radiographers may use this order:

1st	left maxillary premolar
2nd	left maxillary molar
3rd	left mandibular premolar

4th	left mandibular molar
5th	right maxillary premolar
6th	right maxillary molar
7th	right mandibular premolar
8th	right mandibular molar

5. Process the films or scan the phosphor plates or observe the digital images on computer monitor.

COMPETENCY AND EVALUATION

1. Mount the processed radiographs on the simulated film mounts that follow. Secure with a piece of tape placed along the top edge of the radiograph only, so that it may be raised slightly, to allow light underneath for ease of viewing. The use of removable transparent tape will allow the film mount page to be used more than once. (If using digital technology, observe the images on the computer monitor or print out a copy of the images at the direction of your instructor.)

   Note: Use the labial mounting method. (See Laboratory Exercise 6, Film Mounting and Radiographic Landmarks, for details.) The raised portion of the embossed dot is toward you (convex) when placing the radiograph onto the page.

2. Place the page with the mounted radiographs taped to it on a view box and evaluate for acceptability. Circle the ✓ where packet placement, vertical angulation, horizontal angulation, and centering were performed correctly, and the ✗ where performed incorrectly. Identify which error was made by placing an ✗ on the corresponding line.

3. Obtain instructor feedback. Identify which step (packet placement, vertical angulation, horizontal angulation, centering) needs improvement.

4. Repeat Part 1 and Part 2 at the direction of your instructor. The film mount page may be copied to accommodate multiple practice attempts to achieve competency.

5. Having practiced the four steps of packet placement, vertical and horizontal angulation, and centering the x-ray beam, looking back over your self-evaluations, are there any consistencies? Which step do you feel most comfortable with? Which step do you feel needs improvement? What steps can you take to improve? Save these radiographs obtained utilizing the paralleling technique for comparison with the radiographs you expose using the bisecting technique in Laboratory Exercise 5, Periapical Radiographs—Bisecting Technique.

6. Complete the study questions.

Full Mouth Series A

Part 1: Anterior Periapical Radiographs—Maxilla
Mount Films Below

patient's right   patient's left

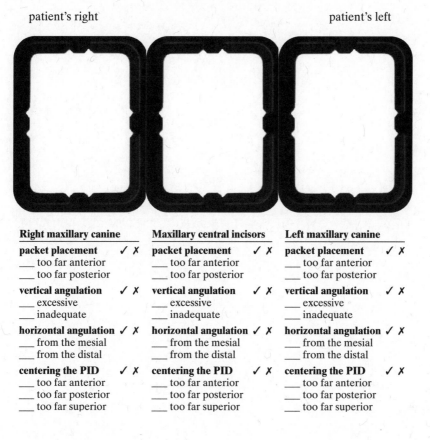

Right maxillary canine			**Maxillary central incisors**			**Left maxillary canine**		
packet placement	✓	✗	**packet placement**	✓	✗	**packet placement**	✓	✗
___ too far anterior			___ too far anterior			___ too far anterior		
___ too far posterior			___ too far posterior			___ too far posterior		
vertical angulation	✓	✗	**vertical angulation**	✓	✗	**vertical angulation**	✓	✗
___ excessive			___ excessive			___ excessive		
___ inadequate			___ inadequate			___ inadequate		
horizontal angulation	✓	✗	**horizontal angulation**	✓	✗	**horizontal angulation**	✓	✗
___ from the mesial			___ from the mesial			___ from the mesial		
___ from the distal			___ from the distal			___ from the distal		
centering the PID	✓	✗	**centering the PID**	✓	✗	**centering the PID**	✓	✗
___ too far anterior			___ too far anterior			___ too far anterior		
___ too far posterior			___ too far posterior			___ too far posterior		
___ too far superior			___ too far superior			___ too far superior		

Full Mouth Series A

Part 1: Anterior Periapical Radiographs—Mandible
Mount Films Below

patient's right   patient's left

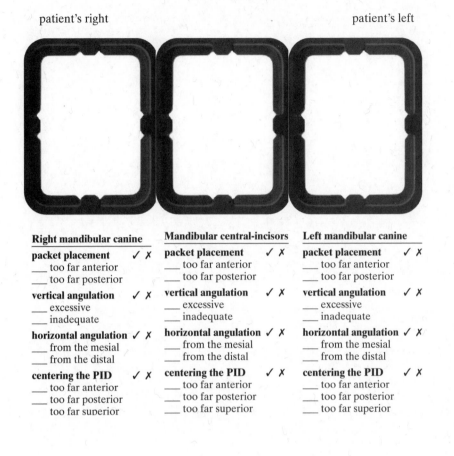

Right mandibular canine		Mandibular central-incisors		Left mandibular canine	
packet placement	✓ ✗	**packet placement**	✓ ✗	**packet placement**	✓ ✗
___ too far anterior		___ too far anterior		___ too far anterior	
___ too far posterior		___ too far posterior		___ too far posterior	
vertical angulation	✓ ✗	**vertical angulation**	✓ ✗	**vertical angulation**	✓ ✗
___ excessive		___ excessive		___ excessive	
___ inadequate		___ inadequate		___ inadequate	
horizontal angulation	✓ ✗	**horizontal angulation**	✓ ✗	**horizontal angulation**	✓ ✗
___ from the mesial		___ from the mesial		___ from the mesial	
___ from the distal		___ from the distal		___ from the distal	
centering the PID	✓ ✗	**centering the PID**	✓ ✗	**centering the PID**	✓ ✗
___ too far anterior		___ too far anterior		___ too far anterior	
___ too far posterior		___ too far posterior		___ too far posterior	
too far superior		___ too far superior		___ too far superior	

NAME _____

Full Mouth Series B
Part 1: Anterior Periapical Radiographs—Maxilla
Mount Films Below

patient's right   patient's left

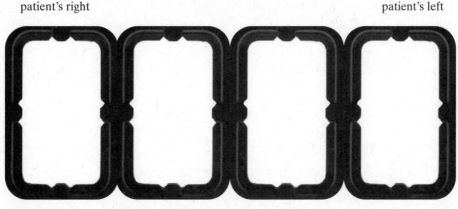

Right maxillary canine	Right maxillary central-lateral incisors	Left maxillary central-lateral incisors	Left maxillary canine
packet placement ✓ ✗	**packet placement** ✓ ✗	**packet placement** ✓ ✗	**packet placement** ✓ ✗
___ too far anterior	___ too far anterior	___ too far anterior	___ too far anterior
___ too far posterior	___ too far posterior	___ too far posterior	___ too far posterior
vertical angulation ✓ ✗	**vertical angulation** ✓ ✗	**vertical angulation** ✓ ✗	**vertical angulation** ✓ ✗
___ excessive	___ excessive	___ excessive	___ excessive
___ inadequate	___ inadequate	___ inadequate	___ inadequate
horizontal angulation ✓ ✗	**horizontal angulation** ✓ ✗	**horizontal angulation** ✓ ✗	**horizontal angulation** ✓ ✗
___ from the mesial	___ from the mesial	___ from the mesial	___ from the mesial
___ from the distal	___ from the distal	___ from the distal	___ from the distal
centering the PID ✓ ✗	**centering the PID** ✓ ✗	**centering the PID** ✓ ✗	**centering the PID** ✓ ✗
___ too far anterior	___ too far anterior	___ too far anterior	___ too far anterior
___ too far posterior	___ too far posterior	___ too far posterior	___ too far posterior
___ too far superior	___ too far superior	___ too far superior	___ too far superior

Full Mouth Series B
Part 1: Anterior Periapical Radiographs—Mandible
Mount Films Below

patient's right   patient's left

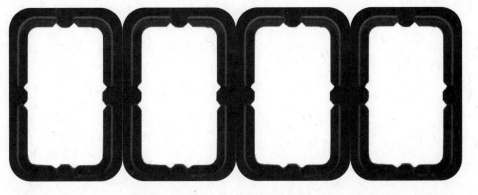

Right mandibular canine	**Right mandibular central-lateral incisors**	**Left mandibular central-lateral incisors**	**Left mandibular canine**
packet placement ✓ ✗	**packet placement** ✓ ✗	**packet placement** ✓ ✗	**packet placement** ✓ ✗
___ too far anterior	___ too far anterior	___ too far anterior	___ too far anterior
___ too far posterior	___ too far posterior	___ too far posterior	___ too far posterior
vertical angulation ✓ ✗	**vertical angulation** ✓ ✗	**vertical angulation** ✓ ✗	**vertical angulation** ✓ ✗
___ excessive	___ excessive	___ excessive	___ excessive
___ inadequate	___ inadequate	___ inadequate	___ inadequate
horizontal angulation ✓ ✗	**horizontal angulation** ✓ ✗	**horizontal angulation** ✓ ✗	**horizontal angulation** ✓ ✗
___ from the mesial	___ from the mesial	___ from the mesial	___ from the mesial
___ from the distal	___ from the distal	___ from the distal	___ from the distal
centering the PID ✓ ✗	**centering the PID** ✓ ✗	**centering the PID** ✓ ✗	**centering the PID** ✓ ✗
___ too far anterior	___ too far anterior	___ too far anterior	___ too far anterior
___ too far posterior	___ too far posterior	___ too far posterior	___ too far posterior
___ too far superior	___ too far superior	___ too far superior	___ too far superior

Full Mouth Series A and B
Part 2: Posterior Periapical Radiographs
Mount Films Below

patient's right side

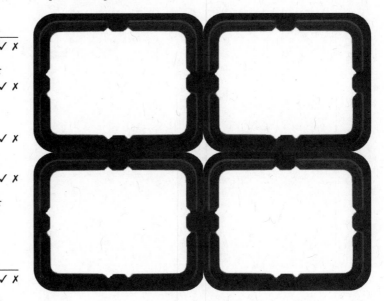

Right maxillary molar

packet placement ✓ ✗
___ too far anterior
___ too far posterior

vertical angulation ✓ ✗
___ excessive
___ inadequate

horizontal angulation ✓ ✗
___ from the mesial
___ from the distal

centering the PID ✓ ✗
___ too far anterior
___ too far posterior
___ too far superior
___ too far inferior

Right maxillary premolar

packet placement ✓ ✗
___ too far anterior
___ too far posterior

vertical angulation ✓ ✗
___ excessive
___ inadequate

horizontal angulation ✓ ✗
___ from the mesial
___ from the distal

centering the PID ✓ ✗
___ too far anterior
___ too far posterior
___ too far superior
___ too far inferior

Right mandibular molar

packet placement ✓ ✗
___ too far anterior
___ too far posterior

vertical angulation ✓ ✗
___ excessive
___ inadequate

horizontal angulation ✓ ✗
___ from the mesial
___ from the distal

centering the PID ✓ ✗
___ too far anterior
___ too far posterior
___ too far superior

Right mandibular premolar

packet placement ✓ ✗
___ too far anterior
___ too far posterior

vertical angulation ✓ ✗
___ excessive
___ inadequate

horizontal angulation ✓ ✗
___ from the mesial
___ from the distal

centering the PID ✓ ✗
___ too far anterior
___ too far posterior
___ too far superior

Full Mouth Series A and B
Part 2: Posterior Periapical Radiographs
Mount Films Below

patient's left side

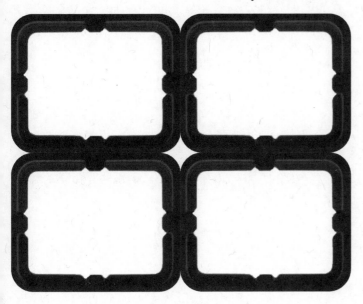

Left maxillary premolar

packet placement   ✓ ✗
___ too far anterior
___ too far posterior

vertical angulation ✓ ✗
___ excessive
___ inadequate

**horizontal
angulation**   ✓ ✗
___ from the mesial
___ from the distal

centering the PID ✓ ✗
___ too far anterior
___ too far posterior
___ too far superior
___ too far inferior

Left maxillary molar

packet placement   ✓ ✗
___ too far anterior
___ too far posterior

vertical angulation ✓ ✗
___ excessive
___ inadequate

**horizontal
angulation**   ✓ ✗
___ from the mesial
___ from the distal

centering the PID ✓ ✗
___ too far anterior
___ too far posterior
___ too far superior
___ too far inferior

**Left mandibular
premolar**

packet placement   ✓ ✗
___ too far anterior
___ too far posterior

vertical angulation ✓ ✗
___ excessive
___ inadequate

**horizontal
angulation**   ✓ ✗
___ from the mesial
___ from the distal

centering the PID ✓ ✗
___ too far anterior
___ too far posterior
___ too far superior

**Left mandibular
molar**

packet placement   ✓ ✗
___ too far anterior
___ too far posterior

vertical angulation ✓ ✗
___ excessive
___ inadequate

**horizontal
angulation**   ✓ ✗
___ from the mesial
___ from the distal

centering the PID ✓ ✗
___ too far anterior
___ too far posterior
___ too far superior

I. Periapical radiographs
   A. Used to diagnose
      1. Suspected periapical condition
      2. Trauma or injury to the teeth
      3. Periodontal involvement
      4. Endodontic therapy
      5. Large carious lesions
      6. Suspected impactions
      7. Unusual eruption pattern, malpositioned or unexplained missing teeth
      8. Unexplained pain
      9. Unusual tooth morphology/color
      10. Evaluation of implants
   B. Types
      1. Anterior
         a. Intraoral image receptor size #1 or size #2 or a combination of both are typically used when exposing anterior periapical radiographs on adults and adolescents after the eruption of the second permanent molars. Anterior periapical radiographs on children with primary dentition (3 to 6 years of age) use intraoral image receptor size #0, and children with transitional (mixed primary and permanent) dentition use size #0 or size #1.
         b. The number and location of placement of image receptors varies among practices.
         c. The long dimension of the image receptor is placed vertically in the oral cavity.
      2. Posterior
         a. Intraoral image receptor size #2 is typically used when exposing posterior periapical radiographs on adults and adolescents after the eruption of the second permanent molars. Posterior periapical radiographs on children with primary dentition (3 to 6 years of age) use image receptor size #0 or size #1, and children with transitional (mixed primary and permanent) dentition use size #1 or size #2.
         b. The number and location of placement of image receptors is standard among practices.
         c. The long dimension of the image receptor is placed horizontally in the oral cavity.
II. Paralleling technique
   A. Image receptor holders
      1. Holder designs range from simple biteblocks to complex instruments that aid in determining the correct alignment of the x-ray beam.
      2. Manufacturers usually offer a set of instruments that can be utilized to expose all regions of the oral cavity.

Figure 4–9 "L"-shaped image receptor holder with an extended biteblock area for use with the paralleling technique.

3. Requirements

a. "L"-shaped holder to provide a stable back for the image receptor (especially film and phosphor plates) to prevent bending while maintaining parallel image receptor-to-tooth relationship (Figure 4–9 ■)

b. Long biteblock area to allow for parallel placement of the image receptor to the long axis of the tooth (Figure 4–9)

B. Principal concepts

1. The white unprinted side of the film packet is placed toward the teeth. PSP plates are labeled to determine front and back sides. The front side of a digital sensor is flat. If using a wired sensor, the wire is attached to the back.

2. The embossed identification dot (film) is positioned away from the area of interest. (Place "dot in the slot" of the film holder to position toward the incisal/occlusal edge and away from the apices of the teeth.)

3. The image receptor is placed parallel to the teeth of interest.

a. The facial tilt of all maxillary teeth (anterior and posterior) requires placing the image receptor an increased distance from the teeth to achieve a parallel relationship between the plane of the image receptor and the long axes of the teeth (Figures 4–10 ■ and 4–11 ■).

b. The facial tilt of mandibular anterior teeth requires placing the image receptor an increased distance from the teeth to achieve a parallel relationship between the plane of the image receptor and the long axes of the teeth (Figures 4–10 and 4–11).

c. Mandibular posterior teeth are very nearly parallel to the midsagittal plane, and therefore the image receptor can usually be positioned close to the lingual surfaces of the teeth in this region and still achieve parallel relationship between the plane of the image receptor and the long axes

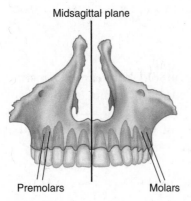

Midsagittal plane

Premolars   Molars

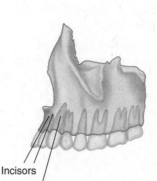

Incisors

Canine

Figure 4–10 All maxillary posterior and anterior teeth tilt outward from the midsagittal plane.

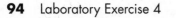

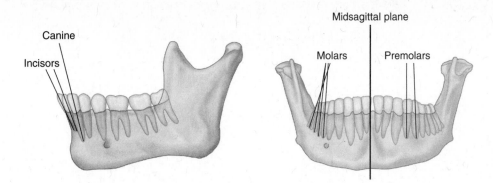

Figure 4–11 The mandibular anterior teeth tilt outward from the midsagittal plane. The mandibular posterior teeth (premolars and molars) are in a position that is parallel to the midsagittal plane (straight upright in the arch), or at a slightly lingual tilt in toward the midsaggital plane.

of the teeth (Figures 4–10 and 4–11). If utilizing the Stabe® film holding device, the bite extension may be removed to shorten the holder in this mandibular posterior region only (Figure 4–12 ■).

    d. A long PID (12 inch/30 cm or 16 inch/41 cm) should be used to minimize distortion that results when the image receptor-to-teeth distance is increased (Figures 4–13 ■ and 4–14 ■).

C. Advantagest
    1. Provides quality images with minimal geometric distortion.
    2. Minimizes the superimposition of adjacent structures.
    3. Has potential for easy standardization of subsequent radiographs.

D. Limitations
    1. Image receptor placement may be uncomfortable for some patients to tolerate.

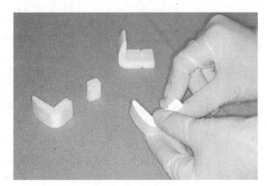

Figure 4–12 This holder's bite extension may be removed and still maintain a parallel relationship between the plane of the image receptor and the long axes of the teeth in the mandibular posterior regions *only*. Using a shortened bite extension in all other regions of the oral cavity requires the use of the bisecting technique. (See Laboratory Exercise 5.)

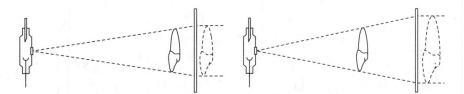

Figure 4–13 Increasing the image receptor-to-tooth distance increases image distortion.

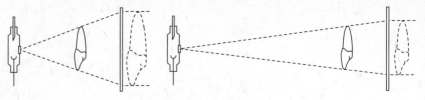

8" Distance   16" Distance

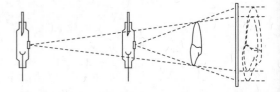

Comparing an 8" distance with a 16" distance

Figure 4–14 Increasing the PID length helps to minimize the distortion resulting from increasing the image receptor-to-tooth distance.

2. True parallel positioning may be difficult for the radiographer to achieve.
3. A long 12 inch/30 cm or 16 inch/41 cm PID often does not come as standard equipment and must be ordered at an additional cost.

III. Full mouth series of periapical radiographs—see Table 4–1
    A. Placement of the image receptor
        1. Image receptor is positioned to image the entire tooth from occlusal/incisal edge to at least 2 mm beyond the apex (root tip).
        2. While there are standard configurations of full mouth series, variations are acceptable and depend on the preference of the practitioner.
    B. Vertical angulation
        1. Determine the up-and-down angulation of the PID. Positive angulation is achieved by pointing the PID down toward the floor. Generally, maxillary periapical radiographs will require a positive vertical angulation, and mandibular periapical radiographs will usually require a negative vertical angulation.
        2. Direct the x-ray beam to intersect the image receptor perpendicularly in the vertical dimension (Figure 4–15 ■). If not using an image receptor holder with an external aiming device, use a tongue blade as an extension of the holder's biteblock; align the vertical angle of the PID parallel to the tongue blade in the vertical dimension (Figure 4–16 ■).

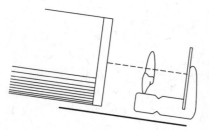

Figure 4–15 Vertical angulation for periapical radiographs should be such that the central rays of the x-ray beam will intersect the image receptor perpendicularly in the vertical dimension. Note the line drawn to indicate that the vertical slant of the PID is parallel to the vertical slant of the extension of the holder.

96 Laboratory Exercise 4

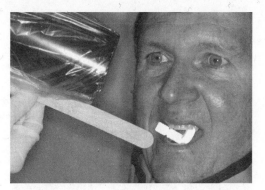

Figure 4–16 Use of a tongue blade acts as a visual aid in determining the correct vertical angulation.

C. Horizontal angulation
   1. Horizontal angulation of the x-ray beam
      a. Determine the side-to-side placement of the PID.
      b. Align the PID such that the central ray of the x-ray beam will intersect the image receptor perpendicularly. Perpendicular alignment of the x-ray beam can be achieved either of two ways:
         1) Direct the central ray of the x-ray beam through a pre-determined interproximal space or directly at the tooth being imaged. Examine the contact points of the patient's teeth to determine the correct horizontal angulation (Figure 4–5).
         2) Using the open end of the PID as the reference point, align such that the open end of the PID is parallel to the image receptor in the horizontal plane. Visualizing the horizontal placement of the PID is easily achieved by using an image receptor holder with an external aiming device (Figure 4–2) or by placing a tongue blade or cotton-tipped applicator across the open end of the PID and rotating the tube head horizontally until the tongue blade indicates that the open end of the PID is parallel to the image receptor (Figure 4–17 ■).
D. Centering the image receptor within the diameter of the x-ray beam
   1. Determine the placement of the image receptor. Use any part of the image receptor holder that is visible outside the mouth as an indication of where the image receptor is located.

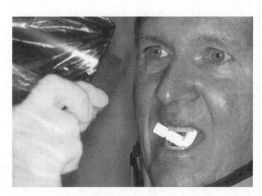

Figure 4–17 Use of a tongue blade acts as a visual aid in determining the correct horizontal angulation.

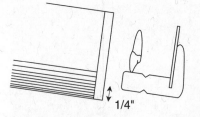
1/4"

Figure 4–18 The PID will be centered over the image receptor when the edge of the PID is aligned into position 1/4 inch below the holder bite extension.

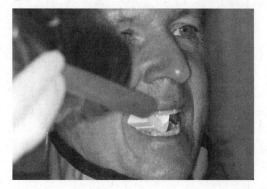

Figure 4–19 Using a tongue blade to visualize correct centering of the x-ray beam over the image receptor.

2. Direct the central rays of the x-ray beam toward the center of the image receptor.
3. Using the image receptor holder as a reference point, align the PID directly over the image receptor. The image receptor will usually be centered in the diameter of the PID when the edge of the PID is positioned 1/4 inch beyond the holder edge (Figure 4–18 ■). Correct positioning of the PID can be achieved by placing the tongue blade as an extension of the PID. No part of the image receptor should be visible beyond the diameter of the PID when extending the tongue blade (Figure 4–19 ■).

IV. Errors
    A. Image receptor placement error
        1. Occurs when the image receptor is not placed correctly intraorally
        2. Results in the appropriate teeth not being recorded
        3. Placed too far anteriorly (Figure 4–20 ■)
        4. Placed too far posteriorly (Figure 4–21 ■)

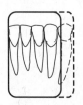

Figure 4–20 A mandibular central-lateral incisors periapical radiograph with image receptor placed too far anteriorly so as not to image the contact between the lateral incisor and the canine.

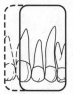

Figure 4–21 A maxillary central-lateral incisors periapical radiograph with image receptor placed too far posteriorly so as not to image the contact between the right and left central incisors.

5. If not positioned (1) perpendicular to the embrasures and (2) parallel to the facial surfaces of the teeth of interest, incorrect horizontal angulation will result. (See horizontal angulation error described later in this section.)

B. Vertical angulation error

1. Occurs when the up-and-down angle of the PID is not set such that the x-ray beam intersects the image receptor perpendicularly in the vertical plane

2. Results in the incisal/occlusal edges or the apices of the teeth not being recorded on the radiograph
   NOTE: If an elongation or foreshortening error is noted (see Laboratory Exercise 5, Periapical Radiographs—Bisecting Technique), then the image receptor was not placed correctly parallel to the long axes of the teeth. When placing the image receptor parallel to the teeth, it is geometrically impossible to get elongation or foreshortening error.

3. Excessive vertical angulation when utilizing the paralleling technique results in the incisal/occlusal edge being cut off the resultant image (Figure 4–22 ■).

4. Inadequate vertical angulation when utilizing the paralleling technique results in the apices' edge being cut off the resultant image (Figure 4–23 ■).

C. Horizontal angulation error

1. Occurs when the side-to-side angulation of the PID is not set such that the x-ray beam will intersect with the image receptor perpendicularly through the embrasures of the teeth of interest; additionally, if the image receptor is not positioned (1) perpendicular to the embrasures and (2) parallel to the facial surfaces of the teeth of interest, the PID cannot be set such that the beam will intersect with the image receptor perpendicularly.

2. Results in superimposition of proximal surfaces of adjacent teeth (overlap error)

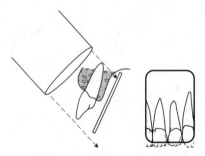

Figure 4–22 When utilizing the paralleling technique, excessive vertical angulation results in incisal/occlusal edges being cut off the image.

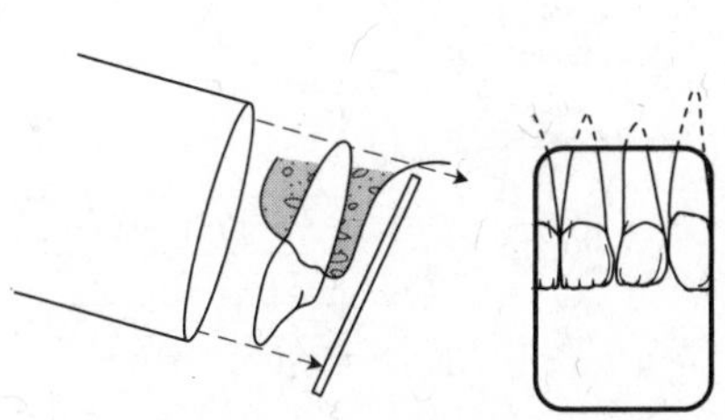

Figure 4–23 When utilizing the paralleling technique, inadequate vertical angulation results in the apices being cut off the image.

3. Occurs when the x-ray beam intersects with the image receptor obliquely from the mesial direction (Figure 4–24 ■)
4. Occurs when the x-ray beam intersects with the image receptor obliquely from the distal direction (Figure 4–25 ■)

D. Centering the x-ray beam over the image receptor error
1. Occurs when the PID is not placed directly over the image receptor
2. Results in an unexposed or clear area (conecut error) recorded on the radiograph
3. Creates a conecut error when the beam is too far toward the anterior (Figure 4–26 ■)
4. Creates a conecut error when the beam is too far toward the posterior (Figure 4–27 ■)
5. Creates a conecut error when the beam is too far toward the superior (Figure 4–28 ■)
6. Creates a conecut error when the beam is too far toward the inferior (Figure 4–29 ■)

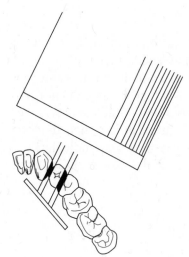

Figure 4–24 When horizontal angulation intersects the image receptor obliquely from the mesial, the most severe overlap occurs in the posterior region of the image.

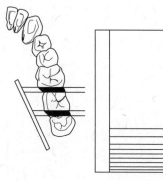

Figure 4–25 When horizontal angulation intersects the image receptor obliquely from the distal, the most severe overlap occurs in the anterior region of the image.

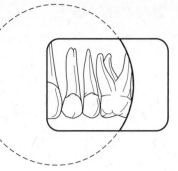

Figure 4–26 When the PID is not centered over the image receptor, an unexposed or clear "conecut" area results. When the conecut is in the posterior section of the image, the PID was positioned too far anteriorly.

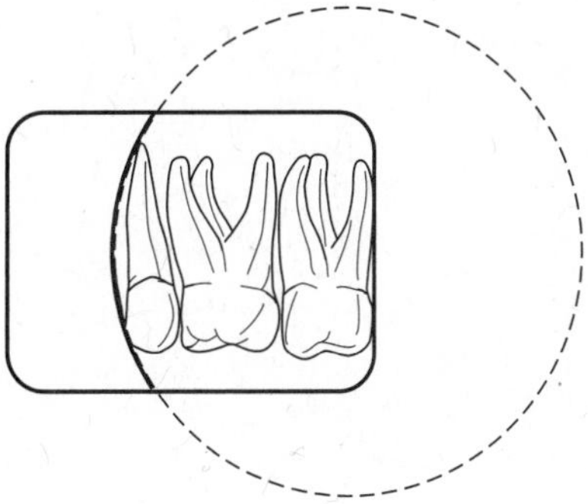

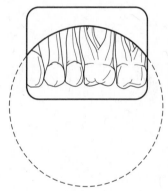

Figure 4–27 When the PID is not centered over the image receptor, an unexposed or clear "conecut" area results. When the conecut is in the anterior section of the image, the PID was positioned too far posteriorly.

Figure 4–28 When the PID is not centered over the image receptor, an unexposed or clear "conecut" area results. When the conecut is in the inferior section of the image, the PID was positioned too far superiorly.

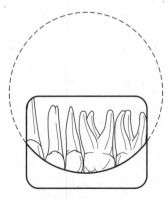

Figure 4–29 When the PID is not centered over the image receptor, an unexposed or clear "conecut" area results. When the conecut is in the superior section of the image, the PID was positioned too far inferiorly.

REFERENCES

American Dental Association Council on Scientific Affairs. (2006). The use of dental radiographs: Update and recommendations. *J. Am. Dent. Assn.,*137, 1304–1312.

Langland, O. E., Langlais, R. P., & Preece, J. W. (2002). *Principles of dental imaging* (2nd ed.). Baltimore, MD: Lippincott Williams & Wilkins, 88.

Thomson, E. M., & Johnson, O. N. (2012). *Essentials of dental radiography for dental assistants and hygienists* (9th ed.). Upper Saddle River, NJ: Pearson.

1. How many posterior periapical radiographs are exposed in a standard adult full mouth series?
   - A. 4
   - B. 6
   - C. 8
   - D. 10

2. Which of the following teeth should be imaged on a mandibular canine periapical radiograph?
   - A. Distal portion of the central incisor, lateral incisor, mesial portion of the canine
   - B. Distal portion of the lateral incisor, canine, mesial portion of the first premolar
   - C. Distal portion of the canine, first premolar, mesial portion of the second premolar
   - D. Distal portion of the first premolar, second premolar, mesial portion of the first molar

3. Which of the following teeth should be imaged on a maxillary premolar periapical radiograph?
   - A. Distal portion of the central incisor, lateral incisor, canine, first premolar, mesial portion of the second premolar
   - B. Distal portion of the lateral incisor, canine, first premolar, second premolar, mesial portion of the first molar
   - C. Distal portion of the canine, first premolar, second premolar, first molar, mesial portion of the second molar
   - D. Distal portion of the second premolar, first molar, second molar, third molar

4. To avoid horizontal overlap error, through which interproximal space should the central ray of the x-ray beam be directed when exposing a mandibular molar periapical radiograph?
   - A. Between the canine and the first premolar
   - B. Between the first premolar and the second premolar
   - C. Between the second premolar and the first molar
   - D. Between the first molar and the second molar
   - E. Between the second molar and the third molar

5. To avoid horizontal overlap error, through which interproximal space should the central ray of the x-ray beam be directed when exposing a maxillary premolar periapical radiograph?
   - A. Between the canine and the first premolar
   - B. Between the first premolar and the second premolar
   - C. Between the second premolar and the first molar
   - D. Between the first molar and the second molar
   - E. Between the second molar and the third molar

6. A mandibular molar periapical radiograph that did not image the entire third molar results from an error made in which of the following?
   A. Packet placement
   B. Vertical angulation
   C. Horizontal angulation
   D. Centering the x-ray beam

7. Referring to question 6, which of the following would correct this error?
   A. Position the image receptor more posteriorly
   B. Increase vertical angulation
   C. Shift the horizontal angulation toward the mesial
   D. Direct the PID more toward the posterior

8. Not recording the apices of the teeth results from an error made in which of the following?
   A. Packet placement
   B. Vertical angulation
   C. Horizontal angulation
   D. Centering the x-ray beam

9. Referring to question 8, which of the following would correct this error?
   A. Position the image receptor more superiorly
   B. Increase vertical angulation
   C. Shift the horizontal angulation toward the distal
   D. Direct the PID more toward the anterior

10. A premolar periapical radiograph that is undiagnostic due to over-lapped interproximal areas is the result of incorrect
    A. Packet placement
    B. Vertical angulation
    C. Horizontal angulation
    D. Centering of the x-ray beam

Periapical Radiographs— Bisecting Technique

INTRODUCTION

The American Dental Association and the American Academy of Oral and Maxillofacial Radiology recommend using the paralleling technique when exposing intraoral radiographs. However, it is not always possible to achieve the ideal parallel image receptor positioning on every patient. Parallelism is difficult to achieve in patients who present with a shallow palatal vault, such as found in children, or when large palatal or mandibular tori are present. When the paralleling technique is not feasible, quality radiographic images may still be acquired if the radiographer has mastered the bisecting technique.

Use of the bisecting technique does not alter the size and number of images required for a full mouth series of radiographs. Additionally, the same four steps of packet placement, vertical angulation, horizontal angulation, and centering the x-ray beam are followed when using either technique. The major differences between the paralleling and bisecting techniques are (1) the image receptor position in relationship to the teeth and (2) the vertical angulation of the PID required to compensate for this position. When using the paralleling technique, the image receptor is placed parallel to the long axis of the tooth; whereas, when employing the bisecting technique, the image receptor is placed as close to the tooth as possible without regard to a parallel relationship. The image receptor may even contact the lingual surfaces of the tooth and oral structures. Because the image receptor and tooth are not parallel, the central rays of the x-ray beam cannot be directed to perpendicularly intersect both the image receptor and the long axis of the tooth. Instead, when using the bisecting technique, the vertical angulation must be directed perpendicular to the imaginary bisector—a plane between the long axes of the image receptor and of the tooth. A general rule is that an increased vertical angulation is required in the bisecting technique over that used for the paralleling technique (Figure 5–1 ■).

Maxilla

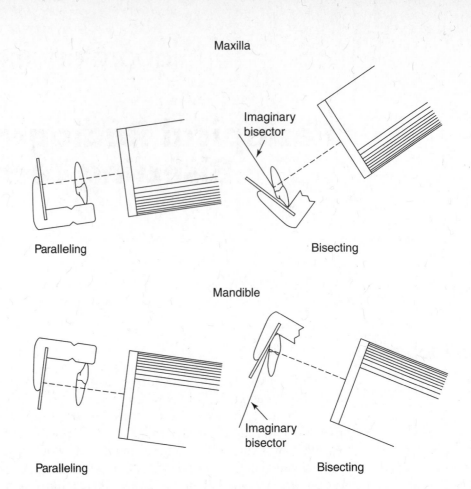

Paralleling

Bisecting

Mandible

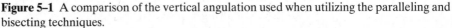

Paralleling

Bisecting

Figure 5–1 A comparison of the vertical angulation used when utilizing the paralleling and bisecting techniques.

This beginning exercise uses the Stabe® (Dentsply Rinn) (Figure 5–2 ■) disposable, polystyrene biteblock film holder, but your instructor may direct you to complete the activity using any of the number of quality image receptor holding devices either for film or photostimuable phosphor (PSP) plates or digital sensors currently on the market (Figures 5–3 ■ and 5–4 ■). The Stabe film holder used to learn the paralleling technique in Laboratory Exercise 3 can be adapted, with a slight modification to be used with both the paralleling and the bisecting techniques. The use of this holder requires a working knowledge of the skills needed to master the bisecting technique, including positioning the image receptor and the PID, especially aligning the vertical and horizontal x-ray beam angulation.

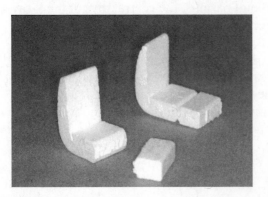

Figure 5–2 Stabe® image receptor holder modified for use with the bisecting technique.

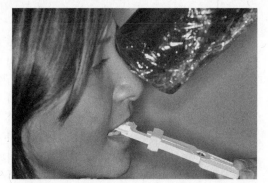

Figure 5–3 Hand-held image receptor holder for use with the bisecting technique.

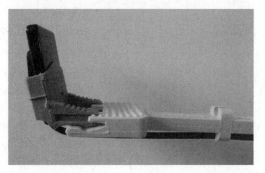

Figure 5–4 Digital sensor image receptor holder for use with the bisecting technique.

Mastering these skills with an understanding of projection geometry will allow you to easily transfer this working knowledge to other periapical image receptor holding devices that do not have an external aiming device.

OBJECTIVES

Following the completion of this lab activity, you will be able to:

1. Alter the Stabe image receptor holder for use with the bisecting technique.

2. Demonstrate proficiency in placing, exposing, and processing anterior and posterior periapical radiographs using the bisecting technique.

3. Critique a full mouth series of intraoral radiographs consisting of anterior and posterior periapicals, for correct (a) placement of the image receptor intraorally, (b) vertical and (c) horizontal angulation of the PID, and (d) direction of the x-ray beam over the entire image receptor.

MATERIALS

Teaching manikin or skull

Lead/lead equivalent apron and thyroid collar

Size #1 and size #2 radiographic films (or digital image receptors)

Periapical film holding device (disposable Stabe or similar device designed for use with the bisecting technique)

Viewbox

Tongue blades

PREPARATION

1. Study the chapter outline to prepare for this laboratory exercise. An understanding of the material presented in the outline is required to complete this activity.

2. Use Table 5–1 to assist you with completing the exercises. Instructor demonstration may enhance knowledge of the laboratory exercise.

3. Prepare radiology operatory. Set up teaching manikin or skull. Ensure that correct "patient" positioning is achieved. To image the maxilla, ensure that the maxillary occlusal plane is parallel to the floor; to image the mandible, ensure that the mandibular occlusal plane is parallel to the floor and the midsagittal plane must be perpendicular to the floor for both maxillary and mandibular exposures.

4. Place lead/lead equivalent apron and thyroid collar over the "patient."

5. The size and/or number of image receptors included in a full mouth series of periapical radiographs varies among practices. The anterior periapical radiographic examination may include the exposure of six, seven, or eight periapical radiographs, whereas the posterior radiographic examination usually remains standard with the exposure of eight periapical radiographs (see Figure 4–3). This exercise will focus on the use of two of the most common full mouth series configurations (see Figures 4–3A and 4–3B).

6. Obtain disposable Stabe periapical film holders or similar device designed for use with the bisecting technique.

7. If using film, orient into the holder so that the embossed identification dot will be placed away from the apices of the teeth. Place the "dot in the slot" of the film holder to position the identification dot of the film packet toward the incisal/occlusal edges of the teeth (see Figure 4–8). If using phosphor plates or digital sensor, orient so that the appropriate side faces the x-ray beam.

8. Start with the anterior exposures. Beginning the examination with the more tolerable anterior placements will help to gain the patient's confidence and cooperation with the procedure.

LABORATORY EXERCISE ACTIVITIES

Part 1: Periapical Radiographs Using the Bisecting Technique—Anterior Region

1. If using *Full Mouth Series A* (see Figure 4–3) for this exercise, you may choose to obtain six size #2 radiographic image receptors or six size #1 radiographic image receptors or a combination of five size #1 and one size #2 radiographic image receptors. If using *Full Mouth Series B* (see Figure 4–3) for this exercise, obtain eight size #1 radiographic image receptors.

2. Place image receptors into the Stabe holder with the long dimension positioned vertically.

3. Check posted exposure factors for the dental x-ray machine prior to placing each image receptor and set for the anterior region; adjust as needed for the maxilla and the mandible and for the canine and the central incisor regions.

TABLE 5–1 Summary of Steps for Acquiring Periapical Radiographs for Adult Patients—Bisecting Technique

Periapical Radiograph	Packet Placement	Vertical Angulation*	Horizontal Angulation	Centering*
Maxillary Central-Lateral Incisors (see Figure 4–3, series configuration A) Use image receptor size #1 or size #2	Center the image receptor to line up behind the central and lateral incisors on both the right and left sides; if using a size #2 image receptor, include the mesial halves of the canines (Figure 5–5 ■).	Direct the central rays of the x-ray beam toward the imaginary bisector between the long axes of the teeth and the image receptor in the vertical dimension; +40 degrees.	Direct the central rays of the x-ray beam perpendicularly through the left and right central incisor embrasure (see Figure 4–5).	Center the image receptor within the x-ray beam; direct the central rays of the x-ray beam toward the center of the image receptor at point near the tip of the nose.
Maxillary Central-Lateral Incisors (see Figure 4–3, series configuration B) Use image receptor size #1	Center the image receptor to line up behind the central and lateral incisors on one side of the mouth; include a portion of the central incisor on the opposite side and a portion of the canine (Figure 5–6 ■).	Direct the central rays of the x-ray beam toward the imaginary bisector between the long axes of the teeth and the image receptor in the vertical dimension; +40 degrees.	Direct the central rays of the x-ray beam perpendicularly through the central incisor and lateral incisor embrasure (see Figure 4–5).	Center the image receptor within the x-ray beam; direct the central rays of the x-ray beam toward the center of the image receptor at a point between the root tips of the central incisor and the canine.
Maxillary Canine (see Figure 4–3, same for both series configurations A & B) Use image receptor size #1 or size #2	Center the image receptor to line up behind the canine; include the distal half of the lateral incisor and the mesial half of the first premolar (Figures 5–5 and 5–6).	Direct the central rays of the x-ray beam toward the imaginary bisector between the long axes of the teeth and the image receptor in the vertical dimension; +45 degrees.	Direct the central rays of the x-ray beam perpendicularly in the horizontal direction at the center of the canine (see Figure 4–5).	Center the image receptor within the x-ray beam; direct the central rays of the x-ray beam toward the center of the image receptor at the root of the canine, near the ala (corner) of the nose.
Maxillary Premolar (see Figure 4–3, same for both series configurations A & B) Use image receptor size #2	Align the anterior edge of image receptor to line up behind the distal half of the canine; include the first and second premolars, first molar, and mesial half of the second molar (Figure 5–7 ■).	Direct the central rays of the x-ray beam toward the imaginary bisector between the long axes of the teeth and the image receptor in the vertical dimension; +30 degrees.	Direct the central rays of the x-ray beam perpendicularly through the first and second premolar embrasure (see Figure 4–5).	Center the image receptor within the x-ray beam; direct the central rays of the x-ray beam toward the center of the image receptor at a point on the ala-tragus line (on the cheek bone) directly below the pupil of the eye.

(continues)

Periapical Radiograph	Packet Placement	Vertical Angulation*	Horizontal Angulation	Centering*
Maxillary Molar (see Figure 4–3, same for both series configurations A & B) Use image receptor size #2	Align the anterior edge of image receptor to line up behind the distal half of the second premolar; include the first, second, and third molars (Figure 5–7).	Direct the central rays of the x-ray beam toward the imaginary bisector between the long axes of the teeth and the image receptor in the vertical dimension; +20 degrees.	Direct the central rays of the x-ray beam perpendicularly through the first and second molar embrasure (see Figure 4–5).	Center the image receptor within the x-ray beam; direct the central rays of the x-ray beam toward the center of the image receptor at a point on the ala-tragus line (on the cheek bone) directly below the outer canthus (corner) of the eye.
Mandibular Central-Lateral Incisors (see Figure 4–3, series configuration A) Use image receptor size #1 or size #2	Center the image receptor to line up behind the central and lateral incisors; if using a size #2 film, include the mesial halves of the canines (Figure 5–5).	Direct the central rays of the x-ray beam toward the imaginary bisector between the long axes of the teeth and the image receptor in the vertical dimension; −15 degrees.	Direct the central rays of the x-ray beam perpendicularly through the left and right central incisor embrasure (see Figure 4–5).	Center the image receptor within the x-ray beam; direct the central rays of the x-ray beam toward the center of the image receptor at a point on the center of the chin 1 in. (2–5 cm) above the lower border of the mandible.
Mandibular Central-Lateral Incisors (see Figure 4–3, series configuration B) Incisors Use image receptor size #1	Center the image receptor to line up behind the central and lateral incisors on one side of the mouth; include a portion of the central incisor on the opposite side and a portion of the canine (Figure 5–6).	Direct the central rays of the x-ray beam toward the imaginary bisector between the long axes of the teeth and the image receptor in the vertical dimension; −15 degrees.	Direct the central rays of the x-ray beam perpendicularly through the central incisor and lateral incisor embrasure (see Figure 4–5).	Center the image receptor within the x-ray beam; direct the central rays of the x-ray beam toward the center of the image receptor at a point on the chin near the central and lateral root tips, 1 in. (2.5 cm) above the lower border of the mandible.

Mandibular Canine (see Figure 4–3, same for both series configurations A & B) Use image receptor size #1 or size #2	Center the image receptor to line up behind the canine; include the distal half of the lateral incisor and the mesial half of the first premolar (Figures 5–5 and 5–6).	Direct the central rays of the x-ray beam toward the imaginary bisector between the long axes of the teeth and the image receptor in the vertical dimension; −20 degrees.	Direct the central rays of the x-ray beam perpendicularly in the horizontal direction at the center of the canine (see Figure 4–5).	Center the image receptor within the x-ray beam; direct the central rays of the x-ray beam toward the center of the image receptor at the center of the root of the canine; 1 in. (2.5 cm) above the inferior border of the mandible.
Mandibular Premolar (see Figure 4–3, same for both series configurations A & B) Use image receptor size #2	Align the anterior edge of image receptor to line up behind the distal half of the canine; include the first and second premolars, first molar, and mesial half of the second molar (Figure 5–7).	Direct the central rays toward the imaginary bisector between the long axes of the teeth and the image receptor in the vertical dimension; −10 degrees.	Direct the central rays of the x-ray beam perpendicularly through the first and second premolar embrasure (see Figure 4–5).	Center the image receptor within the x-ray beam; direct the central rays of the x-ray beam toward the center of the image receptor at a point on the chin 1 in. (2.5 cm) above the lower border of the mandible, directly inferior to the pupil of the eye.
Mandibular Molar (see Figure 4–3, same for both series configurations A & B) Use image receptor size #2	Align the anterior edge of image receptor to line up behind the distal half of the second premolar; include the first, second, and third molars (Figure 5–7).	Direct the central rays of the x-ray beam toward the imaginary bisector between the long axes of the teeth and the image receptor in the vertical dimension; −5 degrees.	Direct the central rays of the x-ray beam perpendicularly through the first and second molar embrasure (see Figure 4–5).	Center the image receptor within the x-ray beam; direct the central rays of the x-ray beam toward the center of the image receptor at a point on the chin 1 in. (2.5 cm) above the lower border of the mandible, directly below the outer canthus (corner) of the eye.

*The patient must be seated in the correct position with the occlusal plane of the arch being imaged parallel to the floor and the midsagittal plane perpendicular to the floor to use the vertical angulation and points of entry recommended in this chart.

Source: Thomson, E. M., & Johnson, O. N. (2012). *Essentials of dental radiography for dental assistants and hygienists* (9th ed.). Upper Saddle River, NJ: Pearson.

Maxillary Central-Lateral Incisors

Maxillary Canine

Mandibular Central-Lateral Incisors

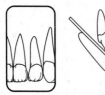

Mandibular Canine

Figure 5–5 Full mouth series A—image receptor placements for anterior periapical radiographs.

Maxillary Central-Lateral Incisors

Maxillary Canine

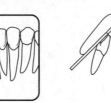

Mandibular Central-Lateral Incisors

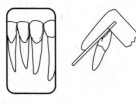

Mandibular Canine

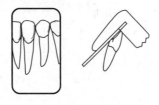

Figure 5–6 Full mouth series B—image receptor placements for anterior periapical radiographs.

Maxillary Premolar

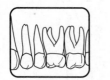

Maxillary Molar

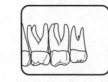

Mandibular Premolar

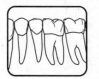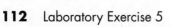

Mandibular Molar

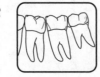

Figure 5–7 Full mouth series A, B, C, D—image receptor placements for posterior periapical radiographs.

4. Place and expose the anterior periapical radiographs in the following order:

Full Mouth Series A (see Figure 4–3A)

1st	right maxillary canine
2nd	maxillary central incisors
3rd	left maxillary canine
4th	left mandibular canine
5th	mandibular central incisors
6th	right mandibular canine

Full Mouth Series B (see Figure 4–3B)

1st	right maxillary canine
2nd	right maxillary central-lateral incisors
3rd	left maxillary central-lateral incisors
4th	left maxillary canine
5th	left mandibular canine
6th	left mandibular central-lateral incisors
7th	right mandibular central-lateral incisors
8th	right mandibular canine

Note: Left-handed radiographers may use this order:

Full Mouth Series A (see Figure 4–3A)

1st	left maxillary canine
2nd	maxillary central incisors
3rd	right maxillary canine
4th	right mandibular canine
5th	mandibular central incisors
6th	left mandibular canine

Full Mouth Series B (see Figure 4–3B)

1st	left maxillary canine
2nd	left maxillary central-lateral incisors
3rd	right maxillary central-lateral incisors
4th	right maxillary canine
5th	right mandibular canine
6th	right mandibular central-lateral incisors
7th	left mandibular central-lateral incisors
8th	left mandibular canine

5. Process the films or scan the PSP plates or observe digital images on computer monitor.

Part 2: Periapical Radiographs Using the Bisecting Technique—Posterior Region

1. Obtain eight size #2 image receptors. All full mouth series configurations on adult patients will most likely use the same standard eight posterior image receptors placements.

2. Place image receptor into the Stabe holder with the long dimension positioned horizontally.

3. Check posted exposure factors for the dental x-ray machine prior to placing each image receptor and set for the posterior region; adjust as needed for the maxilla and the mandible and for the premolar and molar regions.

4. Place and expose the posterior periapical radiographs in the following order:

1st	right maxillary premolar
2nd	right maxillary molar
3rd	right mandibular premolar
4th	right mandibular molar
5th	left maxillary premolar
6th	left maxillary molar
7th	left mandibular premolar
8th	left mandibular molar

   Note: Left-handed radiographers may use this order:

1st	left maxillary premolar
2nd	left maxillary molar
3rd	left mandibular premolar
4th	left mandibular molar
5th	right maxillary premolar
6th	right maxillary molar
7th	right mandibular premolar
8th	right mandibular molar

5. Process the films or scan the phosphor plates or observe the digital images on computer monitor.

COMPETENCY AND EVALUATION

1. Mount the processed radiographs on the simulated film mounts that follow. Secure with a piece of tape placed along the top edge of the radiograph only, so that it may be raised slightly to allow light underneath for ease of viewing. The use of removable transparent tape will allow the film mount page to be used more than once. (If using digital technology, observe the images on the computer monitor or print out a copy of the images at the direction of your instructor.)

Note: Use the labial mounting method. (See Laboratory Exercise 6, Film Mounting and Radiographic Landmarks, for details.) The raised portion of the embossed dot is toward you (convex) when placing the film onto the page.

2. Place the page with the mounted films taped to it on a view box and evaluate for acceptability. Circle the ✓ where packet placement, vertical angulation, horizontal angulation, and centering were performed correctly, and the ✗ where performed incorrectly. Identify which error was made by placing an ✗ on the corresponding line.

3. Obtain instructor feedback. Identify which step (packet placement, vertical angulation, horizontal angulation, centering) needs improvement.

4. Repeat Parts 1 and 2 at the direction of your instructor. The film mount page may be copied to accommodate multiple practice attempts to achieve competency.

5. Compare the periapical radiographs taken utilizing the bisecting technique with those taken using the paralleling technique. (See Laboratory Exercise 4, Periapical Radiographs—Paralleling Technique.) Evaluate the images for diagnostic quality differences and discuss which technique produced the best images. Assess your skills with each of the techniques. Did you find one or the other technique easier to learn? Why? Compare the advantages and disadvantages of the paralleling and the bisecting techniques.

6. Complete the study questions.

Full mouth series A
Part 1: Anterior Periapical Radiographs—Maxilla
Mount Films Below

patient's right   patient's left

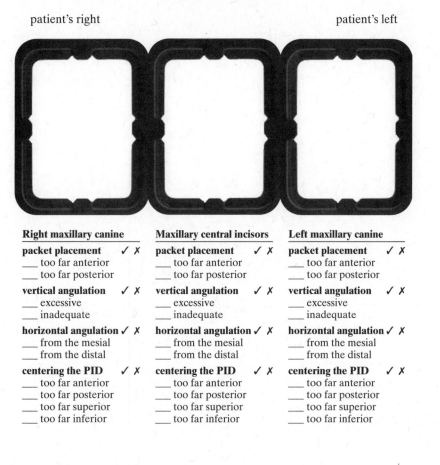

Right maxillary canine	**Maxillary central incisors**	**Left maxillary canine**
packet placement ✓ ✗	**packet placement** ✓ ✗	**packet placement** ✓ ✗
___ too far anterior	___ too far anterior	___ too far anterior
___ too far posterior	___ too far posterior	___ too far posterior
vertical angulation ✓ ✗	**vertical angulation** ✓ ✗	**vertical angulation** ✓ ✗
___ excessive	___ excessive	___ excessive
___ inadequate	___ inadequate	___ inadequate
horizontal angulation ✓ ✗	**horizontal angulation** ✓ ✗	**horizontal angulation** ✓ ✗
___ from the mesial	___ from the mesial	___ from the mesial
___ from the distal	___ from the distal	___ from the distal
centering the PID ✓ ✗	**centering the PID** ✓ ✗	**centering the PID** ✓ ✗
___ too far anterior	___ too far anterior	___ too far anterior
___ too far posterior	___ too far posterior	___ too far posterior
___ too far superior	___ too far superior	___ too far superior
___ too far inferior	___ too far inferior	___ too far inferior

Full mouth series A

Part 1: Anterior Periapical Radiographs—Mandible
Mount Films Below

patient's right   patient's left

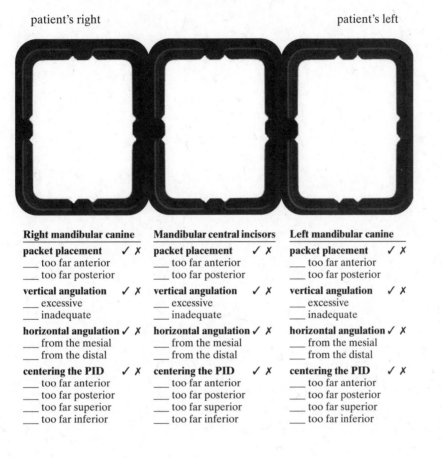

Right mandibular canine	Mandibular central incisors	Left mandibular canine
packet placement ✓ ✗	**packet placement** ✓ ✗	**packet placement** ✓ ✗
___ too far anterior	___ too far anterior	___ too far anterior
___ too far posterior	___ too far posterior	___ too far posterior
vertical angulation ✓ ✗	**vertical angulation** ✓ ✗	**vertical angulation** ✓ ✗
___ excessive	___ excessive	___ excessive
___ inadequate	___ inadequate	___ inadequate
horizontal angulation ✓ ✗	**horizontal angulation** ✓ ✗	**horizontal angulation** ✓ ✗
___ from the mesial	___ from the mesial	___ from the mesial
___ from the distal	___ from the distal	___ from the distal
centering the PID ✓ ✗	**centering the PID** ✓ ✗	**centering the PID** ✓ ✗
___ too far anterior	___ too far anterior	___ too far anterior
___ too far posterior	___ too far posterior	___ too far posterior
___ too far superior	___ too far superior	___ too far superior
___ too far inferior	___ too far inferior	___ too far inferior

Full mouth series B

Part 1: Anterior Periapical Radiographs—Maxilla
Mount Films Below

patient's right   patient's left

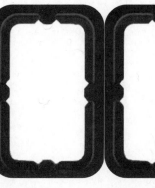

Right maxillary canine	Right maxillary central-lateral incisors	Left maxillary central-lateral incisors	Left maxillary canine
packet placement ✓ ✗	**packet placement** ✓ ✗	**packet placement** ✓ ✗	**packet placement** ✓ ✗
___ too far anterior	___ too far anterior	___ too far anterior	___ too far anterior
___ too far posterior	___ too far posterior	___ too far posterior	___ too far posterior
vertical angulation ✓ ✗	**vertical angulation** ✓ ✗	**vertical angulation** ✓ ✗	**vertical angulation** ✓ ✗
___ excessive	___ excessive	___ excessive	___ excessive
___ inadequate	___ inadequate	___ inadequate	___ inadequate
horizontal angulation ✓ ✗	**horizontal angulation** ✓ ✗	**horizontal angulation** ✓ ✗	**horizontal angulation** ✓ ✗
___ from the mesial	___ from the mesial	___ from the mesial	___ from the mesial
___ from the distal	___ from the distal	___ from the distal	___ from the distal
centering the PID ✓ ✗	**centering the PID** ✓ ✗	**centering the PID** ✓ ✗	**centering the PID** ✓ ✗
___ too far anterior	___ too far anterior	___ too far anterior	___ too far anterior
___ too far posterior	___ too far posterior	___ too far posterior	___ too far posterior
___ too far superior	___ too far superior	___ too far superior	___ too far superior
___ too far inferior	___ too far inferior	___ too far inferior	___ too far inferior

NAME _____

Full mouth series B
Part 1: Anterior Periapical Radiographs—Mandible
Mount Films Below

patient's right   patient's left

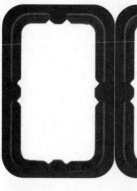

Right mandibular canine	Right mandibular central-lateral incisors	Left mandibular central-lateral incisors	Left mandibular canine
packet placement ✓ ✗	**packet placement** ✓ ✗	**packet placement** ✓ ✗	**packet placement** ✓ ✗
___ too far anterior	___ too far anterior	___ too far anterior	___ too far anterior
___ too far posterior	___ too far posterior	___ too far posterior	___ too far posterior
vertical angulation ✓ ✗	**vertical angulation** ✓ ✗	**vertical angulation** ✓ ✗	**vertical angulation** ✓ ✗
___ excessive	___ excessive	___ excessive	___ excessive
___ inadequate	___ inadequate	___ inadequate	___ inadequate
horizontal angulation ✓ ✗	**horizontal angulation** ✓ ✗	**horizontal angulation** ✓ ✗	**horizontal angulation** ✓ ✗
___ from the mesial	___ from the mesial	___ from the mesial	___ from the mesial
___ from the distal	___ from the distal	___ from the distal	___ from the distal
centering the PID ✓ ✗	**centering the PID** ✓ ✗	**centering the PID** ✓ ✗	**centering the PID** ✓ ✗
___ too far anterior	___ too far anterior	___ too far anterior	___ too far anterior
___ too far posterior	___ too far posterior	___ too far posterior	___ too far posterior
___ too far superior	___ too far superior	___ too far superior	___ too far superior
___ too far inferior	___ too far inferior	___ too far inferior	___ too far inferior

NAME _____

patient's right side

Right maxillary molar

packet placement ✓ ✗
___ too far anterior
___ too far posterior

vertical angulation ✓ ✗
___ excessive
___ inadequate

horizontal angulation ✓ ✗
___ from the mesial
___ from the distal

centering the PID ✓ ✗
___ too far anterior
___ too far posterior
___ too far superior
___ too far inferior

Right maxillary premolar

packet placement ✓ ✗
___ too far anterior
___ too far posterior

vertical angulation ✓ ✗
___ excessive
___ inadequate

horizontal angulation ✓ ✗
___ from the mesial
___ from the distal

centering the PID ✓ ✗
___ too far anterior
___ too far posterior
___ too far superior
___ too far inferior

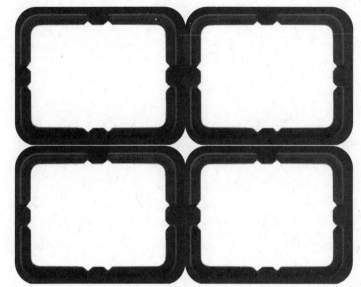

Right mandibular molar

packet placement ✓ ✗
___ too far anterior
___ too far posterior

vertical angulation ✓ ✗
___ excessive
___ inadequate

horizontal angulation ✓ ✗
___ from the mesial
___ from the distal

centering the PID ✓ ✗
___ too far anterior
___ too far posterior
___ too far superior
___ too far inferior

Right mandibular premolar

packet placement ✓ ✗
___ too far anterior
___ too far posterior

vertical angulation ✓ ✗
___ excessive
___ inadequate

horizontal angulation ✓ ✗
___ from the mesial
___ from the distal

centering the PID ✓ ✗
___ too far anterior
___ too far posterior
___ too far superior
___ too far inferior

Full mouth series A and B
Part 2: Posterior Periapical Radiographs
Mount Films Below

patient's left side

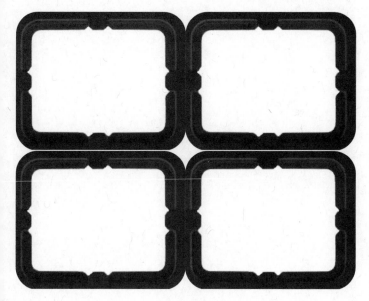

Left maxillary premolar

packet placement ✓ ✗
___ too far anterior
___ too far posterior

vertical angulation ✓ ✗
___ excessive
___ inadequate

**horizontal
angulation** ✓ ✗
___ from the mesial
___ from the distal

centering the PID ✓ ✗
___ too far anterior
___ too far posterior
___ too far superior
___ too far inferior

Left maxillary molar

packet placement ✓ ✗
___ too far anterior
___ too far posterior

vertical angulation ✓ ✗
___ excessive
___ inadequate

**horizontal
angulation** ✓ ✗
___ from the mesial
___ from the distal

centering the PID ✓ ✗
___ too far anterior
___ too far posterior
___ too far superior
___ too far inferior

**Left mandibular
premolar**

packet placement ✓ ✗
___ too far anterior
___ too far posterior

vertical angulation ✓ ✗
___ excessive
___ inadequate

**horizontal
angulation** ✓ ✗
___ from the mesial
___ from the distal

centering the PID ✓ ✗
___ too far anterior
___ too far posterior
___ too far superior
___ too far inferior

**Left mandibular
molar**

packet placement ✓ ✗
___ too far anterior
___ too far posterior

vertical angulation ✓ ✗
___ excessive
___ inadequate

**horizontal
angulation** ✓ ✗
___ from the mesial
___ from the distal

centering the PID ✓ ✗
___ too far anterior
___ too far posterior
___ too far superior
___ too far inferior

I. Bisecting technique
  A. Image receptor holders
    1. The bisecting technique evolved before the development of film holders, so the patient's finger or thumb was used to hold a film packet in place in the oral cavity; no longer acceptable practice because:
       a. Increased patient instruction and cooperation is required.
       b. It is unlikely that the patient can maintain a parallel position between image receptor and teeth.
       c. Movement of the image receptor may occur.
       d. Excessive pressure from the patient's finger or thumb may bend a film packet or photostimuable phosphor (PSP) plate resulting in a distorted image and/or damage to the image receptor.
       e. The finger or thumb will be placed in the path of the primary x-ray beam and incur an unnecessary dose of radiation.
       f. There is no external aiming device to assist with determining the correct angulation.
       g. There could be potential patient objection to placing the fingers in the mouth.
       h. There is the potential to be viewed by the patient as unprofessional and unsanitary.
    2. Requirements
       a. The ability to retain the image receptor in the oral cavity is needed; may or may not have a biteblock backing.
       b. Biteblock backing, if present, is a "V"-shaped slant (Figures 5–4 and 5–8 ■).
       c. Biteblock is short to allow close relationship between image receptor and teeth of interest.
       d. Image receptor placement is as close as possible to or in contact with the lingual surface of the tooth and oral structures, so will not be parallel to the long axes of the teeth (Figure 5–1).
  B. Principal concepts
    1. White unprinted side of the film packet is placed toward the teeth. Photostimuable phosphor (PSP) plates are labeled to determine front and back sides. The front side of a digital sensor is flat. If using a wired sensor, the wire is attached to the back.

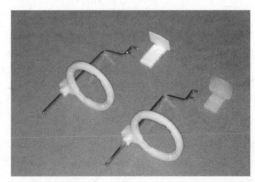

Figure 5–8 Identical image receptor holders with external aiming arm and ring, but with different biteblocks. (Left) biteblock for use with the paralleling technique. (Right) biteblock for use with the bisecting technique.

2. The embossed identification dot (film) is positioned away from the area of interest. (Place dot toward the incisal/occlusal edge and away from the apex of the teeth.)
3. Image receptor is placed as close to the teeth as possible.
   a. Due to the facial tilt the image receptor will not likely be parallel to the long axes of the teeth in the following regions (see Figures 4–10 and 4–11):
      1. Maxillary anterior
      2. Maxillary posterior
      3. Mandibular anterior
   b. The very nearly straight position or slightly lingual tilt of the posterior teeth (molars and premolars) within the mandibular arch allows a close relationship between the lingual surfaces of the teeth and the image receptor to remain parallel (see Figures 4–10 and 4–11).
4. The central ray of the x-ray beam is directed perpendicularly to the imaginary bisector between the image receptor and the long axis of the tooth of interest.
5. Short 8-inch (20.5 cm) or 12-inch (30 cm) PID is required to avoid exaggerating distortion, resulting from lack of parallelism between the plane of the image receptor and the long axes of the teeth.

C. Advantages
1. Image receptor placement may be more comfortable for the patient to tolerate and easier for the operator to achieve. Patients/conditions most likely to benefit from the bisecting technique are:
   a. Low palatal vault
   b. Large torus present
   c. Exaggerated gag reflex
   d. Children (Figure 5–9 ■)
   e. Edentulous regions
2. The image receptor positioning does not require the use of a commercially made holder; it may be stabilized with a custom-made holder such as a hemostat (Figure 5–10 ■) or tongue blade.

D. Limitations
1. Increased image distortion is inherent to the technique. Slight foreshortening or elongation of image usually occurs, especially with maxillary multirooted teeth (Figure 5–11 ■).

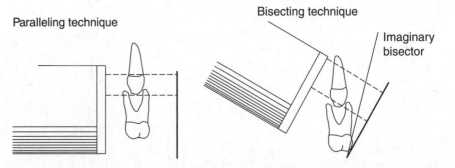

Paralleling technique

Bisecting technique

Imaginary bisector

Figure 5–9 Increased vertical angulation used by the bisecting technique has an added advantage of imaging more of the developing permanent teeth of children.

2. There is increased incidence of superimposition of adjacent structures, especially of the zygoma over the maxillary posterior teeth roots (Figure 5–12 ■).
3. It may increase patient radiation exposure, if using a short 8-inch PID (Figure 5–13 ■).

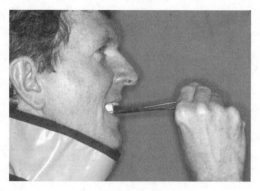

Figure 5–10 Hemostat used as a film holding device for use with the bisecting technique.

Paralleling technique

Bisecting technique

Imaginary bisector

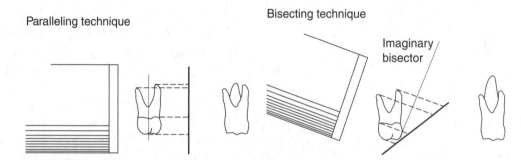
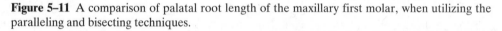

Figure 5–11 A comparison of palatal root length of the maxillary first molar, when utilizing the paralleling and bisecting techniques.

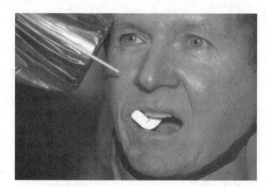

Figure 5–12 Increased vertical angulation for the bisecting technique often superimposes the zygoma over the root of the maxillary first molar on the resultant image.

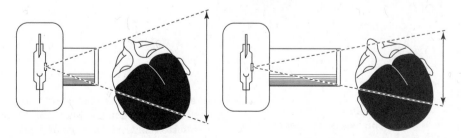

Figure 5–13 A comparison of the diameter of the exiting x-ray beam of radiation exposure with short and long PIDs.

II. Full mouth series of periapical radiographs—see Table 5–1
  A. Placement of the image receptor
    1. The standard configurations of full mouth series of periapical radiographs, with accepted variations, are the same for both the bisecting and paralleling technique (see Figure 4–3).
    2. The primary difference between bisecting and paralleling techniques is that when utilizing the bisecting technique, the image receptor is positioned as close as possible, and not parallel, to the teeth.
  B. Vertical angulation
    1. Generally, the vertical angulation will be increased over that used for the paralleling technique to compensate for a "flatter" position of the image receptor.
    2. Direct the x-ray beam to intersect the imaginary bisector between the plane of the image receptor and the long axis of the tooth perpendicularly (Figure 5–14 ■).
      a. As a visual aid in estimating the imaginary bisector and determining the correct vertical angulation, align the vertical angulation of the PID perpendicular to the image receptor. Make a mental note of this angle. Then realign the PID so that it is now perpendicular to the tooth, and note this angle. Finally, realign the vertical angle of the PID halfway between the two points noted. Reposition the PID perpendicularly to the image receptor, then perpendicularly to the tooth several times, until you can make an accurate judgment of the halfway point (Figures 5–15 ■ and 5–16 ■).
      b. Another technique to help estimate the imaginary bisector location is to align the PID perpendicularly to the plane of the image receptor and note the vertical angulation degrees as indicated on the tube head. Realign the PID perpendicularly to the long axis of the tooth, and note this new setting. Add or subtract to locate the halfway point between these two angles and realign the PID at this angle for the exposure. This procedure is time consuming, but it will be accurate, which is especially important if performing a retake due to estimating the vertical angulation incorrectly the first time.

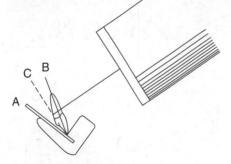

A = Film plane
B = Long axis of the tooth
C = Imaginary bisector

Figure 5–14 Vertical angulation for periapical radiographs using the bisecting technique should be such that the beam will intersect the imaginary bisector between the plane of the image receptor and the long axis of the tooth perpendicularly in the vertical dimension.

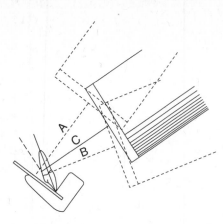

A = Perpendicular to the film plane
B = Perpendicular to the long axis of the tooth
C = Perpendicular to the imaginary bisector

Figure 5–15 Use the two visible planes, the image receptor, and the long axis of the tooth to estimate the invisible imaginary bisector.

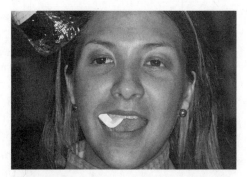

(A)

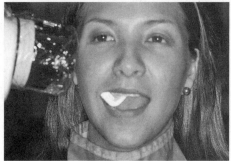

(B)

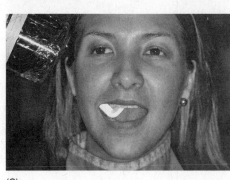

(C)

Figure 5–16 (A) PID is directed perpendicular to the image receptor. (B) PID is directed perpendicular to the long axes of the teeth. (C) PID is directed perpendicular to the imaginary bisector between these two planes.

3. If the patient's head is correctly and precisely positioned, predetermined vertical angulations may be used (Table 5–1).

C. Horizontal angulation—determined in the same manner as for paralleling technique

a. Determine the side-to-side placement of the PID.

b. Align the PID such that the central ray of the x-ray beam will intersect the image receptor perpendicularly. Perpendicular alignment of the x-ray beam can be achieved either of two ways:

1. Direct the central ray of the x-ray beam through a predetermined interproximal space or directly at the tooth being imaged. Examine the contact points of the patient's teeth to determine the correct horizontal angulation (see Figure 4–4).

2. Using the open end of the PID as the reference point, align such that the open end of the PID is parallel to the image receptor in the horizontal plane. Visualizing the horizontal placement of the PID is easily achieved by using an image receptor holder with an external aiming device or by placing a tongue blade or cotton-tipped applicator across the open end and rotating the tube head horizontally until the tongue blade or cotton-tipped applicator, and therefore the open end of the PID, is parallel to the image receptor (Figure 5–16).

D. Centering the image receptor within the diameter of the x-ray beam

1. Determining the location of the center of the image receptor is slightly more difficult with the bisecting technique. Because of a "flatter" position of the image receptor and the increased vertical angulation setting, the radiographer must be skilled in estimating the direction the x-ray beam will travel. Use any part of the holder that is visible outside the mouth as an indication of where the center of the image receptor is located.

2. Direct the central rays of the x-ray beam toward the center of the image receptor.

3. Using the image receptor holder as a reference point, align the PID directly over the image receptor. The image receptor will usually be centered in the diameter of the PID when the edge of the PID is positioned 1/4 inch beyond the holder edge. (Figure 5–17 ■). Correct positioning of the PID can be achieved

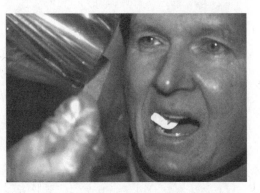

Figure 5–17 Use of a tongue blade acts as a visual aid in determining the correct horizontal angulation.

by placing the tongue blade as an extension of the PID. No part of the image receptor should be visible beyond the diameter of the PID when extending the tongue blade (Figure 5–18 ■).

    4. If the patient's head is correctly and precisely positioned, predetermined points of entry may be used (Table 5–1).

III. Errors

    A. Image receptor placement error

        1. This error results in the appropriate teeth not being recorded.

        2. Errors occur in the same manner as when utilizing the paralleling technique (see Figures 4–20 and 4–21).

        3. If not positioned (1) perpendicular to the embrasures and (2) parallel to the facial surfaces of the teeth of interest, incorrect horizontal angulation will result. (See horizontal angulation error described later in this section.)

    B. Vertical angulation error

        1. This error occurs when the up-and-down angle of the PID is not set such that the x-ray beam intersects the imaginary bisector perpendicularly in the vertical plane.

        2. It results in an elongation or foreshortening error.

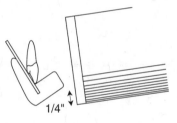

Figure 5–18 X-ray beam will be centered over the image receptor when the edge of the PID is aligned into position 1/4 inch below the extension of the biteblock.

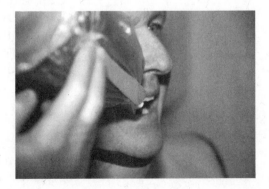

Figure 5–19 Using a tongue blade to visualize correct centering of the x-ray beam over the image receptor.

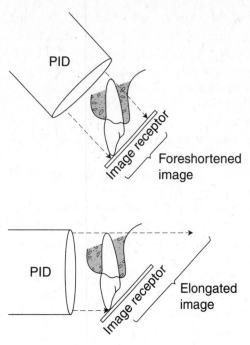

Foreshortened image

Figure 5–20 When utilizing the bisecting technique, excessive vertical angulation results in foreshortening distortion of the image.

Elongated image

Figure 5–21 When utilizing the bisecting technique, inadequate vertical angulation results in elongation distortion of the image.

       3. Excessive vertical angulation when utilizing the bisecting technique results in a foreshortened image (Figure 5–20 ■).

       4. Inadequate vertical angulation when utilizing the bisecting technique results in an elongated image (Figure 5–21 ■).

  C. Horizontal angulation error

       1. This error occurs when the side-to-side angulation of the PID is not set such that the x-ray beam will intersect with the image receptor perpendicularly through the embrasures of the teeth of interest; additionally, if the image receptor is not positioned (1) perpendicular to the embrasures and (2) parallel to the facial surfaces of the teeth of interest, the PID cannot be set such that the beam will intersect with the image receptor perpendicularly.

       2. It results in superimposition of proximal surfaces of adjacent teeth (overlap error).

       3. Errors occur in the same manner as when utilizing the paralleling technique (see Figures 4–24 and 4–25).

  D. Centering the x-ray beam over the image receptor error

       1. The error occurs when the PID is not placed directly over the image receptor.

       2. Errors occur in the same manner as when using the paralleling technique (see Figures 4–26, 4–27, 4–28, and 4–29).

REFERENCES

Langland, O. E., Langlais, R. P., & Preece, J. W. (2002). *Principles of dental imaging* (2nd ed.). Baltimore, MD: Lippincott Williams & Wilkins.

Thomson, E. M., & Johnson, O. N. (2012). *Essentials of dental radiography for dental assistants and hygienists* (9th ed.). Upper Saddle River, NJ: Pearson.

White, S. C., & Pharoah, M. J. (2008). *Oral radiology principles and interpretation* (6th ed.). St. Louis, MO: Elsevier.

1. Through which interproximal space should the central x-ray beam be directed when exposing a maxillary premolar periapical radiograph to achieve accurate horizontal angulation?
   - A. Between the canine and the first premolar
   - B. Between the first premolar and the second premolar
   - C. Between the second premolar and the first molar
   - D. Between the first molar and the second molar
   - E. Between the second molar and the third molar

2. Through which interproximal space should the central x-ray beam be directed when exposing a mandibular molar periapical radiograph to achieve accurate horizontal angulation?
   - A. Between the canine and the first premolar
   - B. Between the first premolar and the second premolar
   - C. Between the second premolar and the first molar
   - D. Between the first molar and the second molar
   - E. Between the second molar and the third molar

3. A maxillary lateral-canine periapical radiograph that did not image the interproximal contact between the lateral incisor and the central incisor results from an error made in which of the following?
   - A. Packet placement
   - B. Vertical angulation
   - C. Horizontal angulation
   - D. Centering the x-ray beam

4. Referring to question 3, which of the following would correct this error?
   - A. Position the image receptor more anteriorly.
   - B. Decrease vertical angulation.
   - C. Shift the horizontal angulation toward the distal.
   - D. Direct the PID more superiorly.

5. Elongated images result from an error made in which of the following?
   - A. Packet placement
   - B. Vertical angulation
   - C. Horizontal angulation
   - D. Centering the x-ray beam

6. Referring to question 5, which of the following would correct this error?
   - A. Place the image receptor farther away from the teeth.
   - B. Increase the vertical angulation.
   - C. Shift the horizontal angulation toward the mesial.
   - D. Direct the PID more inferiorly.

7. Foreshortened images result from an error made in which of the following?
   - A. Packet placement
   - B. Vertical angulation
   - C. Horizontal angulation
   - D. Centering the x-ray beam

8. Referring to question 7, which of the following would correct this error?
   - A. Place the image receptor closer to the teeth.
   - B. Decrease the vertical angulation.
   - C. Shift the horizontal angulation toward the distal.
   - D. Direct the PID more posteriorly.

9. A molar periapical radiograph that is undiagnostic due to overlapped interproximal areas is the result of incorrect
   - A. Packet placement
   - B. Vertical angulation
   - C. Horizontal angulation
   - D. Centering the x-ray beam

10. Evaluate and compare the paralleling and the bisecting techniques. List the advantages and limitations of each. Indicate under what conditions and circumstances you would utilize the paralleling technique and the bisecting technique.

_____

_____

_____

_____

_____

_____

_____

_____

_____

_____

laboratory exercise 6

Mounting and Radiographic Landmarks

INTRODUCTION

Dental radiographs should be correctly oriented according to a standardized method prior to viewing and interpretation. This holds true for both film-based and digital images. Mounted film-based radiographs and correctly orientated digital images minimize misdiagnosis, enhance interpretation, and increase efficiency of the viewing process. Film-based radiographs should be mounted immediately after processing to help protect the films from damage that may result from excessive handling. Digitally acquired images should be immediately positioned into the correct orientation on the computer screen to avoid mixing up the images. A working knowledge of normal radiographic anatomy will help the radiographer correctly mount and orient radiographic images. There are two methods for mounting radiographic images, the labial method, recommended by the American Dental Association, and the lingual method. The dental radiographer should be skilled in utilizing the labial method of film mounting, but must also recognize lingually mounted radiographs and understand the two different orientations.

The purpose of this laboratory exercise is to help you link your knowledge of normal anatomy with the radiographic appearance of common landmarks and to provide practice in mounting intraoral radiographs.

OBJECTIVES

Following completion of this lab activity you will be able to:

1. Differentiate between labial and lingual methods of mounting.

2. Correctly mount a full mouth series of radiographs including bitewings, using the labial method.

3. Locate distinct maxillary and mandibular anatomical landmarks on a radiographic image.

4. Distinguish between a radiolucent and a radiopaque landmark on an intraoral radiograph.

MATERIALS

Scissors

Film mounts

Sample pre-exposed full mouth series

Viewbox

Highlighter pens (six different colors)

PREPARATION

1. Study the chapter outline to prepare for this laboratory exercise. An understanding of the material presented in the outline is required to complete this activity.

2. Your instructor may provide you with samples of patient radiographs in addition to the simulated exercise presented here.

LABORATORY EXERCISE ACTIVITIES

Part 1: Labial Mounting Exercise (FMS Simulation)

1. Cut out the 20 radiographs on the page that follows.

2. Assuming that the embossed dot is raised, i.e., convex, arrange the 20 radiographs on the simulated film mount according to the labial method of film mounting.

3. When you are sure that all 20 radiographs are arranged correctly, secure to the simulated film mount with a piece of tape. Using removable transparent tape will allow you to repeat this exercise or to change the positions of the radiographs as needed.

Part 2: Labial Mounting Exercise (Sample Radiographs)

1. Obtain the sample patient radiographs from your instructor.

2. Obtain the full mouth series film mount from your instructor.

3. Place the sample radiographs on the viewbox and arrange them on the film mount according to the labial method of film mounting.

4. When you are sure that all the radiographs are arranged correctly, secure in the film mount.

Part 3: Anatomic Landmark Identification Exercise

1. When you have completed the mounting exercises, obtain six different colored felt tip highlighter pens.

2. Using a different colored pen for each structure, highlight the following structures on the images of the radiographs you have just mounted on the simulated film mount page.

Maxillary Landmarks

incisive foramen	BLUE
median palatine suture	GREEN
nasal fossa	PINK
maxillary sinus	YELLOW
zygomatic process	PURPLE
maxillary tuberosity	ORANGE

Mandibular Landmarks

lingual foramen	BLUE
genial tubercles	GREEN
inferior border of the mandible	PINK
submandibular fossa	YELLOW
mandibular canal	PURPLE
mental foramen	ORANGE

Part 4: Digital Image Mounting Exercise

1. At the direction of your instructor, open the sample digital patient radiographs to view on the computer monitor. Your instructor has moved the images around the template so that they are not in the correct anatomic positions.

2. Using the computer software, drag-and-drop or cut-and-paste each of the images into the correct positions. Some computer software programs allow you to reverse, flip, or rotate the images as well. Experiment with moving the images around the template.

3. When you are sure that all the images are arranged correctly, save the examination.

COMPETENCY AND EVALUATION

1. List the steps you took to complete the mounting exercises. Discuss why the order of these steps is important. List your own generalizations on how you arrived at the correct arrangement of the radiographs.

2. Explain how a working knowledge of normal radiographic landmarks helped you determine the correct mounting of the radiographs in these exercises.

3. Place the mounted radiographs on the viewbox, or using the digital images displayed on the computer monitor, role-play patient education with a student partner. The student playing the role of the patient should ask you questions regarding the images viewed on the radiographs. For example, the "patient" may point to the large radiolucent area near the maxillary posterior teeth roots and question the

appearance of this region. The student playing the role of radiographer should be able to explain this normal radiographic appearance of the maxillary sinus. Point out to the patient the appearance of the sinus on both the left and right sides. Continue role playing and quiz your partner on the images you see.

4. Complete the study questions.

Part 1: Simulated Radiographs for Labial Mounting Exercise

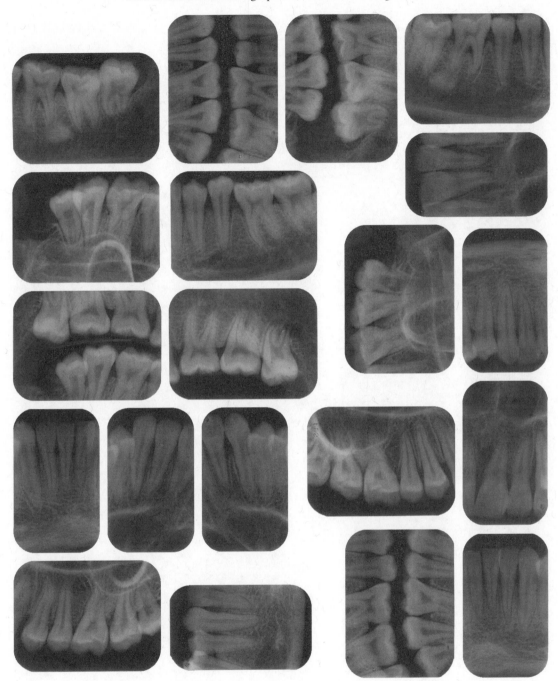

NAME _____

patient's right

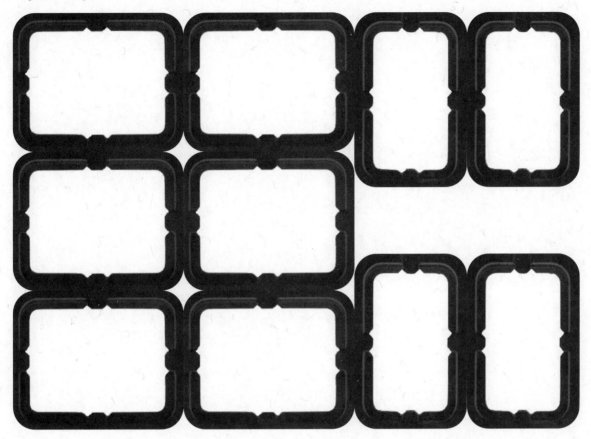

NAME _____

Part 1: Simulated Film Mount for Labial Mounting Exercise

patient's left

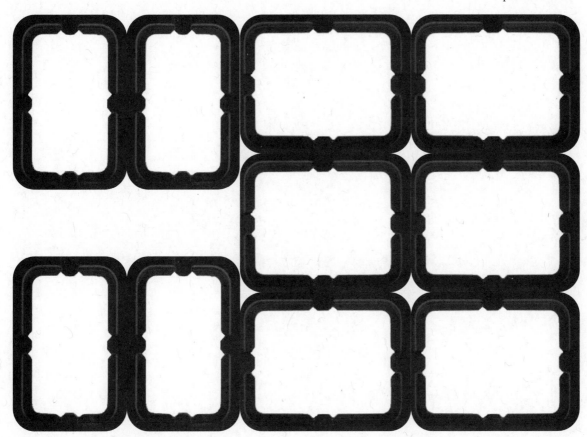

I. Film mounting
  A. Advantages
    1. Minimizes misdiagnosis by orienting the radiograph in its correct anatomical position.
    2. Minimizes confusing the patient's left and right sides.
    3. Maximizes efficiency when radiographs are viewed side by side, allowing easy comparison.
    4. Enhances viewing conditions by masking extraneous light (film-based radiographs.)
    5. Reduces the chance for film damage from excessive handling (film-based radiographs).
    6. Provides a means for documenting patient information, i.e., name, date radiographs were taken, name of radiographer, facility, or practice owner's name.
    7. Aids in charting and documentation of radiographic findings, especially when mounted radiographs and chart diagram represent how the teeth are arranged in the oral cavity.
    8. Aids in patient oral health education and treatment consultations by helping the patient visualize the oral cavity.
  B. Types of film mounts (Figure 6–1 ■)
    1. Mounts may be made of translucent or opaque plastic or vinyl, black or gray cardboard.
    2. Window sizes and configurations and number may vary and can be customized to fit the practice needs.
  C. Film mounting methods
    1. Labial mounting method
      a. It is recommended by the American Dental Association to establish a standard.
      b. It is easily compared with most dental charts, facilitating the transfer of radiographic interpretative findings to the patient record.
      c. Orientation is "from the lips," as though the radiographer is looking at the patient from a position in front (Figure 6–2 ■).
      d. When viewing the radiographs, the patient's right is on the radiographer's left and the patient's left is on the radiographer's right.
      e. The embossed dot located on intraoral film is raised or convex.

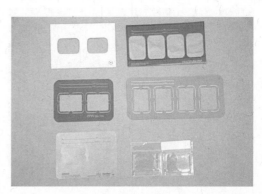

Figure 6–1 A variety of film mounts are currently available.

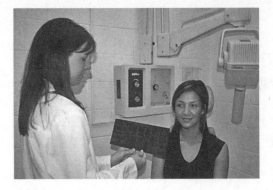

Figure 6–2 With the labial method of mounting radiographs, the orientation is "from the patient's lips."

2. Lingual mounting method
   a. Although still used by some practitioners, the American Dental Association recommends the use of the labial mounting method to establish a standard.
   b. Orientation is "from the tongue," as though the radiographer is looking out from a position inside the oral cavity or from a position behind the patient (Figure 6–3 ■).
   c. When viewing the radiographs, the patient's right is on the radiographer's right, and the patient's left is on the radiographer's left.
   d. The embossed dot located on intraoral film is depressed or concave.
D. Mounting procedure for film-based radiographs (Figure 6–4 ■)
   1. Mount radiographs immediately after processing.
   2. Use clean, dry hands.

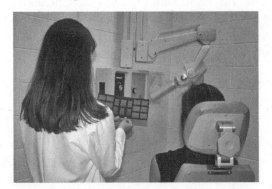

Figure 6–3 With the lingual method of mounting radiographs, the orientation is "from the patient's tongue."

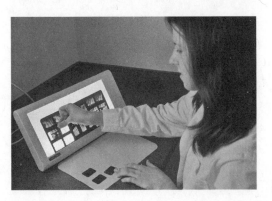

Figure 6–4 Radiographer utilizing a viewbox to mount radiographs.

3. Handle films by the edges only.
4. Place radiographs on a light-colored counter workspace near a viewbox; use a piece of white paper or light-colored tray cover if countertop is dark.
5. Label and date the film mount and place on the viewbox.
6. Arrange all radiographs so the embossed dots are oriented the same direction, i.e., either all raised (convex) when using the labial method or all depressed (concave) when using the lingual method.
7. Separate radiographs by type of projection, i.e., arrange all bitewing radiographs together and all periapical radiographs together.
8. Arrange periapical radiographs by arch imaged, i.e., place all maxillary radiographs together and all mandibular radiographs together.
9. Orient the maxillary periapical radiographs so that the roots are pointing up, and arrange the mandibular periapical radiographs so that the roots are pointing down.
10. Begin placing the radiographs in the labeled film mount.
   a. Place the anterior periapical radiographs.
   b. Place the posterior periapical radiographs.
   c. Place the bitewing radiographs.
E. Mounting procedure for digital radiographs
   1. Direct digital imaging with a solid state sensor
      a. Ensure that the correct window on the template is selected prior to exposure so that the image obtained will automatically be placed into the correct position.
      b. Ensure that the software is set up to match the orientation of the sensor so that the obtained image will not appear upside down in the window.
      c. Using anatomical landmarks, confirm the correct position of the images. Use the computer software to reposition images as needed.
   2. Indirect digital imaging with a photostimuable phosphor (PSP) plate
      a. Use the numbers on the PSP plates or on the infection control barrier envelopes to expose the radiographs in a systematic order so that this same order can be followed when loading the plates into the laser scanner.
      b. Ensure that the PSP plates are placed into the laser scanner in the order that matches the windows of the template.
      c. Using anatomical landmarks, confirm the correct position of the images. Use the computer software to reposition images as needed.
II. Anatomical landmarks
   A. Generalizations that aid in radiographic film mounting
      1. Anterior periapical radiographs (Figure 6–5 ■)
         a. The image receptor is oriented with the longer dimension vertical.
         b. Maxillary anterior teeth are generally wider than mandibular anterior teeth.

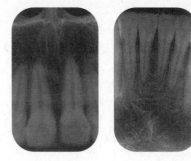

Figure 6–5 Comparison of a maxillary (left) and a mandibular (right) anterior periapical radiograph. Note that the crowns of the maxillary teeth are wider and the roots longer than the mandibular teeth.

    c. Maxillary anterior teeth generally have longer roots than mandibular teeth.

    d. Canines generally have the longest roots when compared with adjacent teeth.

  2. Posterior periapical radiographs (Figure 6–6 ■)

    a. The image receptor is oriented with the longer dimension horizontal.

    b. Mandibular molar teeth usually have two divergent roots with alveolar bone clearly visible in between, whereas maxillary molar teeth have three roots. The superimposition of the maxillary molar palatal root obscures the view of alveolar bone.

    c. Most roots will appear to curve distally.

  3. Bitewing radiographs (Figure 6–7 ■)

    a. The alveolar bone may be more clearly visible between the mandibular molar roots, whereas the maxillary palatal root may obscure the view of alveolar bone.

    b. The occlusal plane or Curve of Spee will appear to slant upward toward the distal, giving the bitewing radiograph a "smile" appearance.

B. Identification of landmarks as an aid in mounting radiographs

  1. Radiopaque landmarks

    a. Dense objects attenuate more of the x-ray beam, leaving less of the beam to strike the image receptor.

    b. Areas appear clear or white to light gray.

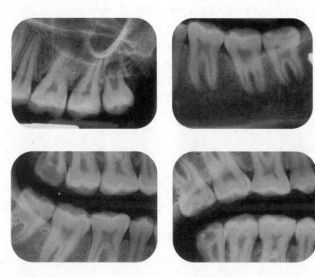

Figure 6–6 Comparison of a maxillary (left) and a mandibular (right) posterior periapical radiograph. Note that the alveolar bone is more clearly visible between the roots of the divergent mandibular teeth, whereas the palatal root of the maxillary molars obscures the view of alveolar bone between the roots.

Figure 6–7 When oriented correctly for mounting (radiograph on left), the occlusal plane (Curve of Spee) will appear to curve upward in a "smile" appearance. Note that when the radiograph is oriented incorrectly (upside down), the occlusal plane will appear to curve downward in a "frown" appearance (radiograph on right).

    c. Radiopaque areas represent dense landmarks such as bony arches, crests, eminences, plates, processes, ridges, septa, spines, tori, tubercles, and tuberosities.

  2. Radiolucent landmarks

    a. Less dense objects allow more of the x-ray beam to penetrate the object and strike the image receptor.

    b. Areas appear black to dark gray.

    c. Radiolucent areas represent less dense landmarks such as openings or depressions in the bone called canals, cavities, fossa, foramina, fissures, meatus, sutures, and sinuses.

C. Landmarks often visible on maxillary anterior radiographs that aid in mounting radiographs (Figures 6–8 ■, 6–9 ■, and 6–10 ■)

  1. Radiopaque

    a. Nasal septum—appears as a vertical, radiopaque bony wall that divides the radiolucent nasal cavity; typically imaged superior to the maxillary central incisors

    b. Anterior nasal spine—appears as a radiopaque triangle-shaped bony protuberance; typically imaged superior to the maxillary central incisors and extending inferior to the nasal septum

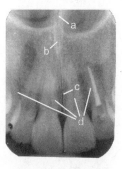

Figure 6–8 (a) Nasal septum, (b) anterior nasal spine, (c) median palatine suture, (d) soft tissue shadow of the nose.

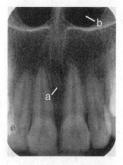

Figure 6–9 (a) Incisive foramen, (b) nasal cavity.

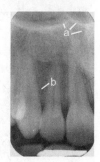

Figure 6–10 (a) Inverted "Y" formation, (b) lateral fossa.

    c. Nasal cavity wall—although the nasal cavity is radiolucent, the dense bony wall of this structure appears as a radiopaque outline typically imaged superior to the maxillary central incisors

    d. Inverted "Y"—a radiopaque landmark created by the intersection of the radiopaque outline of the nasal cavity wall and the radiopaque outline of the maxillary sinus wall, typically imaged near the maxillary canine

    e. Soft tissue shadow of the nose—appears as a radiopaque line often imaged as an arc horizontally across the image

2. Radiolucent

    a. Median palatine suture—appears as a vertical line beginning between the maxillary central incisors; may mimic a fracture line

    b. Incisive (anterior palantine) foramen—appears as a radiolucent oval between the maxillary central incisors

    c. Nasal fossa (cavity)—appears as paired radiolucent ovals superior to the maxillary central incisor roots

    d. Lateral fossa—appears as a diffuse radiolucency between the roots of the maxillary lateral incisor and canine

D. Landmarks often visible on maxillary posterior radiographs that aid in mounting radiographs (Figures 6–11 ■ and 6–12 ■)

1. Radiopaque

    a. Zygomatic process (arch) of the maxilla—appears as a radiopaque "U" or "J" shape inferior to or superimposed over the maxillary first molar roots

    b. Zygoma (cheekbone)—appears as a thick radiopaque band extension of the zygomatic process; often superimposed across the maxillary molar roots

    c. Maxillary tuberosity—appears as a raised bony alveolar ridge in the most distal region of the maxilla, yet still remaining on the maxillary bone

    d. Hamulus (hamular process)—appears as a radiopaque spine projecting inferior and distal to the maxillary tuberosity

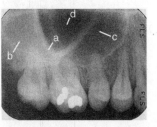

Figure 6–11 (a) Zygomatic process, (b) zygoma, (c) maxillary sinus, (d) nutrient canal.

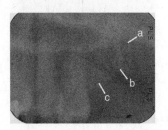

Figure 6–12 (a) Lateral pterygoid plate, (b) hamular process, (c) maxillary tuberosity.

e. Lateral pterygoid plate—appears distal to the maxilla; a radiolucent line (suture) may be visible separating the lateral pterygoid plate from the maxilla

2. Radiolucent

    a. Maxillary sinus—appears as a large radiolucent area extending from the canine to the posterior region of the maxilla, outlined by a dense radiopaque bony wall; appears in almost every radiographic projection of the posterior maxilla

    b. Nutrient canal—appears as a faint radiolucent line extending horizontally across the maxillary sinus on some patients

E. Landmarks often visible on mandibular anterior radiographs that aid in mounting radiographs (Figures 6–13 ■, 6–14 ■, and 6–15 ■)

1. Radiopaque

    a. Mental ridge—appears as a sloping radiopaque band inferior to or superimposed over the roots of the mandibular anterior teeth; the two sides of the ridge may actually resemble an inverted "V" when viewed on the mandibular central incisor periapical radiograph

    b. Genial tubercles—radiopaque spines, often appearing in a circle located inferior to the mandibular central incisors

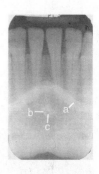

Figure 6–13 (a) Mental ridge, (b) genial tubercles, (c) lingual foramen.

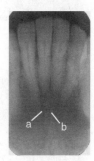

Figure 6–14 (a) Nutrient canals, (b) mental fossa.

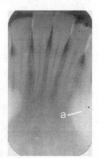

Figure 6–15 (a) Mandibular tori.

      c. Mandibular tori—appear on some patients as round radiopaque "cotton balls" located inferior to or superimposed over the mandibular teeth

      d. Inferior border of the mandible—if the vertical angulation is increased, the inferior border of the mandible may be recorded as a dense, radiopaque band; the area inferior to this image appears radiolucent or black, representing the space beyond the mandible

      e. Soft tissue shadow of the lip—appears as a horizontal radiopaque line, often visible across the anterior teeth

  2. Radiolucent

      a. Lingual foramen—appears as a small radiolucency in the center of the circle formed by the genial tubercles

      b. Mental fossa—appears as a diffuse radiolucency superimposed across the roots of the mandibular anterior teeth; often mimicking a cyst or other apical pathosis

      c. Nutrient canal—appears as a vertical radiolucent line on some patients

F. Landmarks often visible on mandibular posterior radiographs that aid in mounting radiographs (Figures 6–16 ■, 6–17 ■, and 6–18 ■)

  1. Radiopaque

      a. Mylohyoid ridge—appears as a radiopaque line extending from the molar region anteriorly and inferiorly; usually appears inferior to or superimposed over the mandibular molar roots

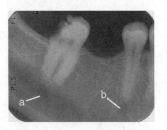

Figure 6–16 (a) Oblique ridge, (b) mylohyoid ridge, (c) inferior border of the mandible.

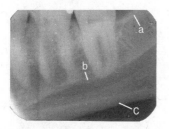

Figure 6–17 (a) Submandibular fossa, (b) mental foramen.

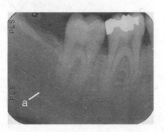

Figure 6–18 (a) Mandibular canal.

b. Oblique ridge—appears as a radiopaque line extending from the ramus anteriorly and inferiorly; usually appears superimposed over the mandibular molar roots
   c. Distinguishing the mylohyoid ridge and the oblique ridge when both landmarks are visible:
      1) The mylohyoid ridge appears more inferior, usually extends further anteriorly, and is not likely to be superimposed over the mandibular molar roots.
      2) The oblique ridge appears more superior and is usually superimposed over the molar teeth.
   d. Inferior border of the mandible—if the vertical angulation is increased, the inferior border of the mandible may be recorded as a dense, radiopaque band; the area inferior to this image appears radiolucent or black, representing the space beyond the mandible
   e. Mandibular tori—appear on some patients as round radiopaque "cotton balls" located inferior to or superimposed over the mandibular teeth
2. Radiolucent
   a. Mental foramen—appears as a circular radiolucency near the mandibular second premolar root; often mimicking periapical pathosis
   b. Mandibular canal—appears as a radiolucent horizontal canal outlined by parallel radiopaque lines (canal walls) traversing the mandible; the mandibular canal appears inferior to or superimposed over the mandibular posterior teeth roots
   c. Submandibular fossa—appears as a large radiolucency in the posterior body of the mandible inferior to the mylohyoid ridge
   d. Nutrient canal—appears as a vertical radiolucent line on some patients

REFERENCES

Haring, J. I., & Lind, L. J. (1993). *Radiographic interpretation for the dental hygienist.* St. Louis, MO: Saunders/Elsevier.

Langlais, R. P. (2003). *Exercises in oral radiography and interpretation* (4th ed.). St. Louis, MO: Saunders/Elsevier.

Thomson, E. M., & Johnson, O. N. (2012). *Essentials of dental radiography for dental assistants and hygienists* (9th ed.). Upper Saddle River, NJ: Pearson.

1. Each of the following is an advantage of mounting radiographs EXCEPT one. Which one is the EXCEPTION?
   A. Eliminates the need for duplicate radiographs
   B. Reduces the chance for film damage
   C. Aids in charting and documentation
   D. Minimizes misdiagnosis

2. Which of the following methods of mounting radiographs is recommended by the American Dental Association?
   A. Labial method
   B. Lingual method

3. Which of the following indicates the labial method of mounting radiographs?
   A. Embossed dot is concave, viewer orientation is facing the patient.
   B. Embossed dot is convex, viewer orientation is facing the patient.
   C. Embossed dot is concave, viewer orientation is facing in the same direction as the patient
   D. Embossed dot is convex, viewer orientation is facing in the same direction as the patient

4. Which of the following is NOT true when using generalizations as an aid to mounting radiographs?
   A. Most roots curve mesially.
   B. The occlusal plane curves upward into a "smile" appearance.
   C. Maxillary anterior teeth are wider then mandibular anterior teeth.
   D. Mandibular molars have two roots while maxillary molars have three.

5. Which of the following would appear radiolucent on a radiograph?
   A. Anterior nasal spine
   B. Genial tubercles
   C. Maxillary sinus
   D. Mental ridge

6. Which of the following would appear radiopaque on a radiograph?
   A. Incisive foramen
   B. Mylohyoid ridge
   C. Mental foramen
   D. Median palatine suture

7. Each of the following would be likely to appear on a maxillary anterior radiograph EXCEPT one. Which one is the EXCEPTION?
   A. Lateral fossa
   B. Nasal septum
   C. Incisive foramen
   D. Maxillary tuberosity

8. Each of the following would be likely to appear on a maxillary posterior radiograph EXCEPT one. Which one is the EXCEPTION?
   - A. Hamulus
   - B. Nasal fossa
   - C. Zygomatic process
   - D. Lateral pterygoid plate

9. Each of the following would be likely to appear on a mandibular anterior radiograph EXCEPT one. Which one is the EXCEPTION?
   - A. Mental foramen
   - B. Genial tubercles
   - C. Lingual foramen
   - D. Mental ridge

10. Each of the following would be likely to appear on a mandibular posterior radiograph EXCEPT one. Which one is the EXCEPTION?
    - A. Mental fossa
    - B. Submandibular fossa
    - C. Mandibular canal
    - D. Oblique ridge

laboratory exercise 7

Identifying and Correcting Radiographic Errors

INTRODUCTION

The valuable role dental radiographs play in the assessment and diagnosis of oral conditions must be balanced with the potential risk that radiation exposure carries. Exposure to dental radiation should be kept to a minimum. Retake radiographs needed when errors are made that compromise radiographic quality double patient exposure; increase the radiation dose to the same tissue area; increase the dose rate, since most retakes are taken without a recovery period between exposures; require additional patient consent; reduce patient confidence in the oral health care professional's ability to provide care; and decrease productivity. Errors that do not result in retakes still diminish the usefulness of the radiograph. Images that lack proper density, contrast, and clarity reduce the value of the radiograph and jeopardize diagnosis. Reduced quality radiographs are also a practice management risk should they be required as evidence in legal matters.

The increasing use of digital imaging with its reduction in radiation exposure over film-based radiography should not contribute to careless attention to technique or an attitude of easy retakes. The benefits from radiation dose reduction should be passed along to the patient, and not become the basis for making the decision to simply take an undiagnostic radiograph over, "because the dose is small." Additionally, the ability to increase or decrease digital image density with computer software will not compensate for a severely under- or overexposed radiograph and should not be relied upon to make up for exposure errors.

Radiographic errors can be organized into three categories: technique errors, processing errors, and image receptor handling errors. Errors may be made singly or as a result of a combination of errors. Often a technique error may mimic a processing error and vice versa. Awareness of the more common errors can help the radiographer take steps to prevent the errors from occurring in the first place. Recognition of pitfalls will also help the radiographer to evaluate images for quality. And, most important, knowledge of the cause of the error and its corrective action will aid the radiographer in taking the appropriate steps to prevent additional retake radiographs.

In this exercise you will have the opportunity to create radiographic errors, allowing you to study the error's cause and corrective action. The purpose of this exercise is to provide an opportunity to identify radiographic pitfalls and to develop the problem-solving skills necessary to recommend the appropriate corrective action.

OBJECTIVES

Following completion of this lab activity, you will be able to:

1. Identify characteristics of a quality radiographic image.

2. Recognize common radiographic technique, processing, and image receptor handling errors.

3. Recommend appropriate corrective action when confronted with a poor quality radiograph.

MATERIALS

Teaching manikin or skull

Lead/lead equivalent apron and thyroid collar

Size #1 and size #2 radiographic films, digital image receptor, and photostimuable phosphor (PSP) plate

Periapical and bitewing image receptor holders

Manual processing tanks and chemicals or rapid/chairside processing cups and chemicals

Thermometer, timer, film rack

Viewbox

PREPARATION

1. Study the chapter outline to prepare for this laboratory exercise. An understanding of the material presented in the outline is required to complete this activity.

2. Prepare radiology operatory. Set up teaching manikin or skull. Ensure that correct "patient" positioning is achieved, that is, occlusal plane parallel to the floor, midsagittal plane perpendicular to the floor.

3. Place lead/lead equivalent apron and thyroid collar over the "patient."

4. Instructor demonstration may enhance knowledge of the laboratory exercise.

LABORATORY EXERCISE ACTIVITIES

Part 1: Technique Error—Comparing Accidental White Light Exposure and No Exposure Errors

The most basic skill of radiographic error identification is being able to determine if a radiographic film has been overexposed, as is the case when a film is accidentally exposed to white light or not exposed at all. The ability to distinguish between which error causes the radiographic image to be too dark, or black, and which error causes the radiographic image to be too light, or clear, provides the basis for determining more complex errors. In this activity you will purposely produce these two errors and then be challenged to determine which is which.

1. Obtain two size #2 films.
2. DO NOT EXPOSE THESE FILMS TO RADIATION.
3. Go to the darkroom, secure the door, turn off the overhead white light, and turn on the safelight.
4. Open and process one of the films in the usual manner.
5. Next, turn on the overhead white light and open and process the other film under unsafe white light conditions.

Part 2: Technique Error—Demonstration of Reversed Image Receptor Error—Film

Several errors can cause a radiographic image to appear too light or underexposed. Prior to taking corrective action, the cause of the light image should be determined. Without determining the cause of the error, inappropriate corrective action may result in a repeat error. Therefore, the first step in determining the cause of a light image is to view the film carefully for the image of the pattern embossed into the lead foil of the film packet. The purpose of this activity is to demonstrate how this pattern gets imaged onto the radiograph when the film packet is positioned into the oral cavity backward.

1. Obtain one each of a size #2 and a size #1 radiographic film packet.
2. Prepare to expose the maxillary central incisors periapical radiograph. Place the size #2 film packet in the film holding device backward. Place the film packet so that the printed, colored side is facing the x-ray beam. This is backward or reversed placement of the film packet.
3. Check posted exposure settings and place and expose the maxillary central incisor periapical radiograph using the paralleling technique.
4. Repeat steps 2 and 3 with the size #1 film packet.
5. Process the two films.

Part 3: Technique Error—Demonstration of Reversed Image Receptor—Digital Sensor or Photostimuable Phosphor (PSP) Plate

Solid state digital sensors and photostimuable phosphor (PSP) plates have front and back sides. Placing these digital image receptors into the oral cavity backward creates a unique error. The purpose of this activity is to assist you in recognizing when backward image receptor placement has occurred.

1. Obtain one each of a size #2 digital sensor and/or PSP plate.

2. Prepare to expose the maxillary central incisors periapical radiograph. Place the size #2 image receptor in the holding device backward. Examine the image receptor to determine which side should be positioned to face the x-ray beam and reverse the placement.

3. Check posted exposure settings and place and expose the maxillary central incisor periapical radiograph using the paralleling technique.

4. Digital sensor: Observe the image on the computer monitor. PSP plate: Remove from the holder and pass into the laser scanning device. Observe the image on the computer monitor.

Part 4: Technique Error—Double Exposure Error—Film and Photostimuable Phosphor (PSP) Plate

Double exposure can be a difficult error to recognize. This is especially true when the two images are very similar to each other, as is the case when a bitewing radiograph is double exposed with another bitewing radiograph of a different region. The purpose of this activity is to provide the opportunity to view the unique image that results from a double exposure error.

1. Obtain one size #2 radiographic film packet and/or one size #2 phosphor plate.

2. Prepare to expose the right premolar and the right molar bitewing radiographs. Place the image receptor in the holding device for exposure of the right premolar bitewing radiograph first.

3. Check posted exposure settings and place and expose the right premolar bitewing radiograph.

4. Next, using the same image receptor, check posted exposure settings and place and expose the right molar bitewing radiograph.

5. Process the film and/or place the PSP plate into the laser scanner and observe the image on the computer monitor.

Part 5: Processing Error—Effect of Developer Time on Radiographic Density

In addition to technique errors, mistakes made during the processing steps can also render a radiograph undiagnostic and result in a retake exposure. The radiographer should possess a working knowledge of the effects processing chemicals have on the radiographic image to be prepared to solve darkroom problems. The purpose of this activity is to determine the results of over- and underdevelopment.

1. Obtain two size #2 radiographic film packets.

2. Prepare to expose the maxillary central incisors periapical radiograph. Place one of the film packets in the holding device. Place the other film aside for use later.

3. Check posted exposure settings and place and expose the maxillary central incisors periapical radiograph using the paralleling technique, using the first film.

4. Process the exposed film manually. Follow the steps for manual processing (see Laboratory Exercise 1 outline), but double the standard developing time. For example, if the standard developing time based on the developer temperature is 5 minutes, then leave the film in the developer for 10 minutes for this experiment. The fixing and washing times are not altered.

5. While the first film is developing, repeat step 3 using the second film.

6. Process this second film manually. Follow the steps for manual processing (see Laboratory Exercise 1 outline), but reduce the standard developing time by one-half. For example, if the standard developing time based on the developer temperature is 5 minutes, then leave the film in the developer for 2.5 minutes for this experiment. The fixing and washing times are not altered.

Part 6: Processing Error—Fixer First Error

Whether processing manually or utilizing an automatic film processor, the steps for film processing must be performed in order. The developer and the fixer each play a specific role in the processing procedure. Reversing the procedure order can cause disastrous effects. The purpose of this activity is to demonstrate the effect of placing the exposed radiographic film into the fixer first during manual processing and/or incorrectly filling the first compartment of an automatic processor with fixer instead of developer.

1. Obtain one size #2 radiographic film packet.

2. Prepare to expose the maxillary central incisor periapical radiograph. Place the film packet in the holding device.

3. Check posted exposure settings and place and expose the maxillary central incisor periapical radiograph using the paralleling technique.

4. Manually process the film by placing it into the fixer first. Then rinse, place in the developer and complete with the washing step.

Part 7: Processing Error—Inadequate Washing

The radiographer should possess the ability to identify when the processing solutions are not functioning at peak potential. To develop this skill, a working knowledge of the function of each solution is needed. The purpose of this activity is to demonstrate the effect of inadequate washing on the resultant radiographic image.

1. Obtain one size #2 radiographic film packet.
2. Prepare to expose the maxillary central incisor periapical radiograph. Place the film packet in the holding device.
3. Check posted exposure settings and place and expose the maxillary central incisor periapical radiograph using the paralleling technique.
4. Turn off the main water valve to the automatic processor or empty the wash water container on a closed system processor.
5. Process the film.
6. Examine the radiograph after securing to the simulated film mount and record today's date. Two weeks from today, re-examine the radiograph.

Part 8: Film Handling Error—Bending the Image Receptor Prior to Exposure

Careful handling of film and of photostimuable phosphor (PSP) plates is needed to avoid damage to the image receptor that is likely to compromise the image quality. Bending or creasing a film packet or PSP plate can occur accidentally when placing into or removing from the image receptor holder. The purpose of this activity is to demonstrate what effect bending the film will have on the resultant image. (You will use an intraoral film for this exercise, but will not damage a PSP plate.) Awareness of the results may help the radiographer understand why film bending to fit the oral cavity is contraindicated.

1. Obtain one size #2 radiographic film packet.
2. Prepare to expose the maxillary central incisor periapical radiograph. Prior to placing the film packet in the holding device, crease one of the corners.
3. Check posted exposure settings and place and expose the maxillary central incisor periapical radiograph using the paralleling technique.
4. Process the film.

Part 9: Photostimuable Phosphor (PSP) Plate Handling Error—Exposing the PSP Plates to Bright Light

Photostimuable phosphor technology is considered indirect digital imaging, requiring a laser scanning step after exposure to produce an image on a computer monitor. After exposure, PSP plates require protection from bright light exposure if not placed immediately into the laser scanning device. This exercise will demonstrate the result of careless handling of the plates following exposure.

1. Obtain two size #2 PSP plates.

2. Prepare to expose the maxillary central incisors periapical radiograph. Place one of the PSP plates in the holding device. Place the other PSP plate aside for use later.

3. Check posted exposure settings and place and expose the maxillary central incisors periapical radiograph using the paralleling technique, using the first PSP plate.

4. Set the exposed PSP plate face up on the counter.

5. Repeat step 3 with the second PSP plate.

6. Set this second PSP plate face up with one of the corners covering approximately half of the first PSP plate.

7. Leave both plates on the counter undisturbed for approximately 10 minutes.

8. After approximately 10 minutes, place both PSP plates into the laser scanner and observe the images on the computer monitor

Part 10: A Problem-Solving Activity

For the past several weeks you have been practicing intraoral radiographic techniques for the first time. As a beginning radiographer, you have probably created some errors along the way. This is your chance to use these mistakes as a valuable teaching tool. Choose one of your radiographic errors and mount this film on the simulated film mount page that follows. Submit this error page with your attached radiograph to your instructor who will number and post one error page from everyone in the class. The challenge to you will be to view each of the posted errors and (1) identify the cause and (2) suggest a corrective action. If you do not have an error to submit for this activity, purposely create one now. Use the outline that follows to select an error to create.

COMPETENCY AND EVALUATION

1. Mount the processed radiographs on the simulated mount pages that follow. Secure with a piece of tape placed along the top edge of the radiograph only, so that it may be raised slightly, to allow light underneath for ease of viewing. Using removable transparent tape will allow the film mount page to be used more than once.
   NOTE: Use the labial mounting method. (See Laboratory Exercise 6, Film Mounting and Radiographic Landmarks, for details.) The raised portion of the embossed dot is toward you (convex) when placing the radiograph onto the page.

2. Examine the resultant radiographic images in each of the first nine activities of this exercise. Based on your results, summarize the following in your own words:

Part 1: How would you explain the effect of accidental white light exposure compared with no exposure of the image receptor? Why is one dark and the other clear?

Part 2: How can you tell when a radiographic film packet has been placed in the patient's mouth backward?

Part 3: How can you tell when a digital sensor or PSP plate has been placed in the patient's mouth backward?

Part 4: Describe the unique appearance of accidentally exposing the same image receptor twice.

Part 5: Describe the effects of over and under developing on the radiographic image density. Explain the cause of the increased/ decreased density.

Part 6: Describe the effect of placing the film into the fixer solution first. Explain the cause of this effect.

Part 7: What effect did inadequate washing have on the radiograph on the day you processed the film? What effect was noticeable two weeks later? Why do you think this occurred? What do you predict will happen to the radiograph as time passes?

Part 8: What effect will bending the film have on the resultant image?

Part 9: Describe the unique appearance of the radiographic images produced by the PSP plates that were exposed to bright light. Explain the cause of this appearance.

3. When your instructor has posted the errors collected from your class, view each of the samples and write out your answer to these questions:
   a. What is the error created here?
   b. What is the corrective action?

NOTE: Your answers should be technical and not obvious. For example, do not answer "blank film" for a radiograph that is clear. "No exposure" or "unexposed" would be a more appropriate answer. Likewise, do not answer "expose the film" as the obvious corrective action. Think about how the radiograph could have resulted in no exposure. It is possible that the film did not get exposed because the radiographer mixed up the exposed film packets with the unexposed film packets while taking a full mouth series. Therefore, a more appropriate answer for the corrective action would be "follow an organized and systematic method of exposing film packets during the radiographic procedure."

There may be more than one correct answer for each error. In our example above, we suggested a technique error for the clear or blank film. A clear film could also result from the processing error of placing the film in the fixer first. Again, your corrective action should not state the obvious, "place the film in the developer first." Instead, think about how this error could have resulted. A more appropriate response would be "label the processing chemical tanks," to prevent placing the film into the fixer first.

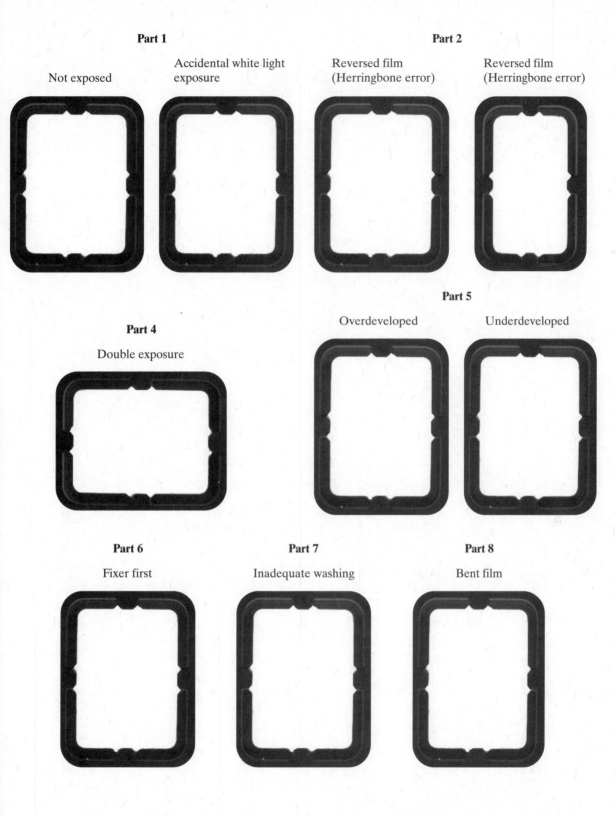

Part 1

Not exposed

Accidental white light exposure

Part 2

Reversed film (Herringbone error)

Reversed film (Herringbone error)

Part 4

Double exposure

Part 5

Overdeveloped

Underdeveloped

Part 6

Fixer first

Part 7

Inadequate washing

Part 8

Bent film

NAME _____

Error Identification

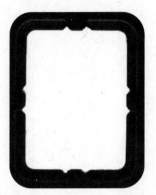

Submit this error page to your instructor to number and post for Part 10 of this exercise.

I. Characteristics of diagnostic quality dental radiographs
   A. General characteristics
      1. An accurate representation of the area being radiographed
      2. Exhibits correct density (not too light/too dark)
      3. Free of image distortion (magnification/elongation/foreshortening)
      4. No overlapping of the interproximal areas
      5. No conecut error
      6. Free of technical, processing, and image receptor handling errors
   B. Bitewing radiographs
      1. Images correct teeth (see Table 2–1)
      2. Equal representation of the maxillary and mandibular arches recorded
      3. Occlusal plane straight or slightly curved upward
      4. Most distal contact imaged (third molars if erupted)
   C. Periapical radiographs
      1. Images correct teeth (see Table 4–1)
      2. At least 2 mm of alveolar bone recorded beyond the apices of the teeth
      3. At least 2 mm margin recorded between the edge of the radiograph and the crowns of the teeth
      4. Each tooth imaged at least once, preferably twice in a full mouth series of periapical radiographs
      5. The embossed dot (on film-based radiographs) positioned at the incisal/occlusal edge of the radiograph

II. Radiographic errors
   A. Dark images
      1. Resulting from overexposure
         a. Errors
            1) Exposure time or impulse setting too high
            2) Milliamperage setting too high
            3) Kilovoltage setting too high
            4) Accidental white light exposure
         b. Corrective actions
            1) Post exposure setting chart for reference.
            2) Consult the exposure setting chart prior to each exposure.
            3) Adjust the exposure settings based on the thickness/density of the subject/object being imaged.
            4) Locate the overhead white light switch away from the working area to prevent accidentally turning on the white light in the darkroom.
      2. Resulting from overdeveloping
         a. Errors
            1) Developing time too long
            2) Developer temperature too warm
            3) Overconcentrated chemical mix
            4) Contamination of the developer solution with fixer chemistry

b. Corrective actions
   1) Consult the time/temperature chart prior to manually processing films.
   2) Allow adequate time for automatic processor to adjust temperature prior to processing films.
   3) Take the temperature of the developer prior to manually processing films.
   4) Secure the developer thermostat in the automatic processing unit.
   5) Carefully mix concentrated chemicals with the appropriate ratio of water prior to use.
   6) Handle replenishing chemicals carefully to avoid contamination (Figure 7–1 ■).

B. Partially dark radiographs/black artifacts
  1. Resulting from overexposure
   a. Errors
    1) Accidental white light exposure
    2) Static electricity exposure
   b. Corrective actions
    1) Carefully remove film packet from the holding device so as not to tear the outer protective wrap, allowing white light to enter and expose the film.
    2) Allow the film to completely enter the automatic processor prior to turning on the white light.
    3) Secure the light-tight cover of the manual processing tanks prior to turning on the white light.
    4) Slowly unwrap film packets to avoid creating a static discharge of white light.
    5) Use a humidifier to reduce dry conditions conducive to static electricity.
    6) Place an antistatic treated grounding device in the darkroom such as commercially available antistatic sprays or clothes dryer fabric sheets to discharge static prior to film handling.
  2. Resulting from overdevelopment
   a. Errors
    1) Developer contamination
    2) Overlapped films during processing (fixer not in contact with film emulsion)
    3) Roller marks

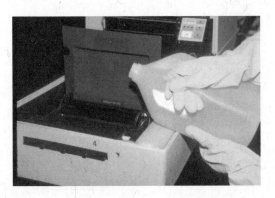

Figure 7–1 Using the tank cover to separate the developer and fixer chemicals during replenishing helps to avoid chemical contamination that can result in poor quality radiographs.

b. Corrective actions
1) Maintain cleanliness in the darkroom to avoid chemical contamination of films prior to processing.
2) When loading films into the automatic processor, use alternating feeder slots or wait approximately 10 seconds between each film to avoid overlapping; if fixer does not contact the emulsion, that portion of the film will fade to black when removed from the processor and exposed to white light.
3) Do not overload manual processing tanks with several film processing racks to avoid film contact.
4) Properly maintain processor, replenishing and replacing chemistry according to manufacturer's recommendations.
   a) As exhausted chemistry breaks down, the solutions become slick, causing films to become stuck on the automatic processing rollers.
   b) As the rollers turn, the films do not advance, but slide on the turning rollers, which creates black horizontal bands of overdeveloped areas on the films.

3. Resulting from incorrect handling of image receptor
a. Errors
1) Film or PSP plate bending/creasing
2) Embossed dot incorrectly positioned during packet placement in the oral cavity (Figure 7–2 ■)
3) Black paper stuck to the film emulsion
4) Glove powder contamination
5) Excessive wetting of PSP plate with disinfectant
6) Damaged/broken digital sensor wire

b. Corrective actions
1) Carefully handle image receptors, especially when placing into holders.
2) Use an edge cushion or smaller-sized image receptor to ease placement intraorally, rather than bend or crease to fit the oral cavity.
3) Place the embossed dot away from the area of interest, i.e., place at the occlusal/incisal edge when placing the film for periapical radiographs.
4) Immediately upon removal from the oral cavity, wipe excess saliva from the film packet (especially paper-wrapped packets) to prevent saliva from seeping into the packet causing the black paper to adhere to the film (see Figure 8–7).

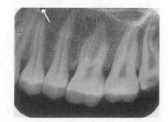

Figure 7–2 When placed near the area of interest such as the apex of the tooth, the embossed dot may obscure pertinent diagnostic information.

5) Carefully unwrap film packets to completely separate the film from the outer plastic/paper wrap, the black paper insert, and the lead foil sheet.

6) Follow infection control protocol to avoid touching the unprocessed films or PSP plates with gloves or hands contaminated with glove powder residue. (See Laboratory Exercise 8, Infection Control and Student Partner Practice.)

7) Do not pull or twist the digital sensor cord; store flat, avoid tangling.

C. Light images
  1. Resulting from underexposure
    a. Errors
      1) Exposure time or impulse setting too low
      2) Milliamperage setting too low
      3) Kilovoltage setting too low
      4) Distance between the open end of the PID and the patient's skin too great (Figure 7–3 ■)
      5) Backward placement of the film packet intraorally so that the x-ray beam must penetrate the lead foil prior to reaching the film
        a) Placing the film packet so that the colored side with the printed information is facing the x-ray beam (Figure 7–4 ■)

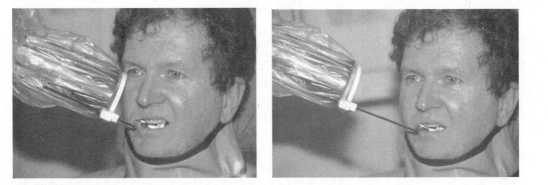

Figure 7–3 (Left) Correct position of the PID in relation to the external aiming device of the image receptor holder. (Right) This incorrect position will result in an underexposed radiographic image.

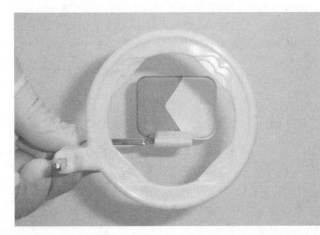

Figure 7–4 Backward film packet placement. Note that the back of the film packet will be incorrectly exposed first, resulting in a light image.

b) Lack of knowledge about which is the front side of the film packet

c) Hurried, unorganized film packet placement

d) Using an unfamiliar film holding device

b. Corrective actions

1) Check for a reversed film packet placement as evidenced by the presence of a tire-track or block pattern recorded onto the image (Figure 7–5 ■). Sometimes referred to as herringbone error after the herringbone pattern produced by early commercial film products.

a) When in doubt about the correct side of the film packet, read the information written on the colored side that states "opposite side toward tube" or similar wording.

b) Be systematic and organized when placing and exposing radiographs.

c) Become familiar with the film holding device before using it to avoid placing the film incorrectly.

2) Post exposure setting chart near the x-ray machine control panel for reference.

3) Consult the exposure setting chart prior to each exposure.

4) Adjust the exposure settings based on the thickness/density of the subject/object.

5) Keep the exposure button depressed throughout the duration of the exposure.

6) Place the open end of the PID as close to the patient's skin as possible without touching. If using an image receptor holder with an external aiming device, slide the aiming ring in toward the patient, until it almost contacts the skin (Figure 7–3).

2. Resulting from underdevelopment

a. Errors

1) Developing time too short

2) Developer temperature too cool

3) Underconcentrated chemical mix

4) Exhausted chemicals

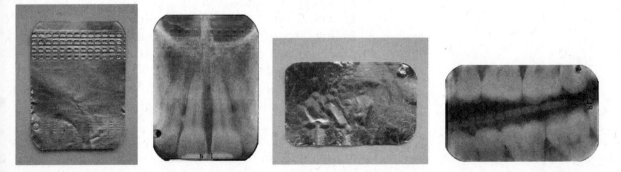

Figure 7–5 These embossed patterns will be imaged when the lead foil faces the x-ray beam, resulting in herringbone error. Note the different patterns, depending on the film size and manufacturer.

b. Corrective actions
   1) Consult the time/temperature chart prior to manually processing films.
   2) Allow adequate time for automatic processor to adjust temperature prior to processing films.
   3) Check the temperature of the developer prior to manually processing films.
   4) Check fluid level of the developer in the automatic processor to ensure that the films will be submerged throughout the processing procedure.
   5) Carefully mix concentrated chemicals with the appropriate ratio of water prior to use.
   6) Replenish and change chemistry according to manufacturer's recommendations.

3. Resulting from incorrect handling of PSP plates
   a. Error
      1) Exposure to bright light
      2) Left face up on counter top too long
   b. Corrective actions
      1) Use containment box available from manufacturer to protect PSP plates from bright light if not scanning immediately after exposure
      2) Ensure that sensitive side of the PSP plate faces down and is protected from light if allowed to remain on countertop

D. Clear/blank film
   1. Resulting from no exposure
      a. Errors
         1) Confusing the image receptor with one that had been exposed
         2) Not turning on the power to the x-ray machine
         3) Placing intraorally, but neglecting to align the PID toward the image receptor
         4) Placing the digital sensor or PSP plate backwards into the oral cavity
         5) Other digital signals in the area interfering with wireless digital sensor transmission of data to the computer
      b. Corrective actions
         1) Develop a systematic routine for exposing radiographs.
         2) Label exposed image receptors and keep separated from unexposed ones during the procedure.
         3) Follow an organized and systematic routine; perform prealignment of the PID prior to placing the image receptor intraorally.
         4) Become familiar with the digital sensor or PSP plate before using it to avoid placing the image receptor incorrectly.
         5) Eliminate the nearby use of other devices that generate electronic signals that interfere with wireless digital sensor technology.

2. Resulting from incorrect processing
   a. Errors
      1) Placing the film into the fixer solution first, allowing the fixer to remove the undeveloped silver halide crystals from the emulsion
      2) Automatically processing the film with no developer solution in the tank
      3) Extended time in the fixer or water during processing, causing the emulsion to separate from the film base
   b. Corrective actions
      1) Label the processing tanks to prevent confusing the developer and fixer tanks.
      2) Read developer and fixer container labels to prevent pouring developer into the fixer tank and fixer into the developing tank during replenishing.
      3) Ensure that the automatic processor is adequately filled with developer solution.
      4) Ensure that the developer tank drain plug is secure to prevent solution from draining out.
      5) Do not leave films overnight in the fixer solution or wash water.
3. Resulting from incorrect handling of digital sensors and PSP plates
   a. Errors
      1) Damaged wire to digital sensor
      2) Computer program not activated to capture the exposure data
      3) Exposing PSP plates to bright light erases the image
   b. Corrective actions
      1) Do not pull or twist the digital sensor cord; store flat and avoid tangling.
      2) Develop the skills to operate the computer software to activate the digital imaging program.
      3) Use containment box to protect PSP plates from bright light if not scanning immediately after exposure.
      4) Ensure that sensitive side of the PSP plate faces down and is protected from light if allowed to remain on countertop.
E. Partially clear/blank film/white artifacts
   1. Resulting from no/underexposure
      a. Errors
         1) Conecut error
            a) Not centering the image receptor in the path of the x-ray beam
            b) Incorrect assembly of the image receptor holding device, causing the x-ray beam to be centered incorrectly
      b. Corrective actions
         1) Use a holding device that aids in centering the image receptor in the path of the x-ray beam.
         2) Learn the appropriate assembly of the image receptor holding device prior to using it.

2. Resulting from incorrect handling of image receptor and ineffective patient management
   a. Errors
      1) Foreign object recorded on the radiograph
      2) Scratched film emulsion or PSP plate
      3) Crimp mark from film or PSP plate bending prior to exposure
      4) Dead pixels (digital sensors) may not be recording all data
      5) Partial image missing, often evident as a straight line indicating a computer software or setup problem
   b. Corrective actions
      1) Ask patient to remove metal objects in or near the oral cavity.
         a) Glasses
         b) Partial/full denture
         c) Orthodontic retainer
         d) Facial jewelry (tongue, lip, nose piercing adornments)
      2) Assess the use of the lead/lead equivalent thyroid collar for some patients. When used on children or adults with a short neck-to-shoulder relationship, the lead/lead equivalent thyroid collar may be in the path of the primary beam.
      3) Carefully handle films, especially when clipping to manual film processing racks, to avoid scratched emulsion, and PSP plates, especially when loading in to the laser scanner.
      4) Avoid overlapping or allowing films to contact each other or the sides of the manual processing tanks to avoid torn emulsion.
      5) Avoid bending the film packet or PSP plate. To increase patient comfort during placement of the image receptor, utilize an edge cushioning product or a smaller size. (See Laboratory Exercise 9, Patient Management and Student Partner Practice, Figures 9–2 and 9–3)
      6) Test sensor to determine the need for replacement if dead pixels no longer capture the image data.
      7) Set up the computer program again or have digital software serviced to eliminate glitch that may contribute to not recording a portion of the image.
F. Green artifacts
  1. Resulting from incorrect or inadequate film processing
   a. Errors
      1) Films become overlapped or stuck together in the automatic processor, preventing chemicals from reaching the emulsion.
      2) Double film packets that are not separated prior to processing prevent chemicals from reaching the emulsion.
      3) Attaching a film to the top clip on the manual processing film rack in combination with a reduced developer and a reduced fixer solution level in both manual processing tanks (caused by evaporation or extended use) may prevent chemicals from reaching a portion of the film (Figure 7–6 ■).

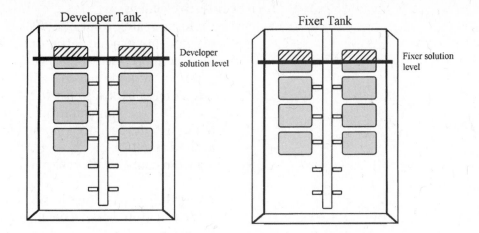

Figure 7–6 When evaporation of chemistry from manual processing tanks prevents both developer and fixer from reaching the film emulsion, the resulting error is a green, unprocessed portion of the film.

        4) Weak or exhausted fixer cannot adequately clear the film.

    b. Corrective actions

        1) When loading films into the automatic processor, use alternating feeder slots or wait approximately 10 seconds between each film to avoid overlapping, preventing processing chemicals from reaching the film emulsion.

        2) Carefully separate double film packets prior to loading onto manual film processing racks or into the automatic processor.

        3) Monitor the solution levels.

        4) Replenish solutions regularly.

        5) Do not attach films to the top manual processing film rack.

  G. Brown artifacts

    1. Resulting from incorrect film processing

      a. Error—Inadequate film rinsing and washing

      b. Corrective actions

        1) Allow the films to wash for the full recommended time.

        2) Ensure that the water to the running water bath (for manual processing and the water supply to the automatic processing unit) is turned on. Ensure that the rinse water bottles are full on closed-system automatic processors.

  H. Fogged image (film) or radiographic noise (digital imaging)

    1. Resulting from exposure to damaging conditions

      a. Errors

        1) Inadequate safelighting

        2) Old, expired film

        3) Accidental exposure of the image receptor to stray radiation, excessive heat and humidity, chemical fumes, or white light

        4) Exposure settings that are extremely low. When switching from film-based radiography to digital imaging, there is a tendency to set the exposure factors too low, resulting in noise (similar in appearance to film fog).

      b. Corrective actions

         1) Perform quality assurance tests to determine adequacy of safelighting in the darkroom and efficacy of film.

         2) Protect image receptors, especially those that have just exposed, from the causes of film fog/radiographic noise.

         3) Use correct exposure settings. After setting at manufacturer's recommendations, evaluate the images to determine the need for varying the settings to obtain the desired result.

  2. Resulting from contact with contaminated solutions

      a. Errors

         1) Using the same paddles to stir solutions

         2) Not cleaning and drying the manual processing film racks before using again.

         3) Careless handling of processing chemistry during replenishment.

         4) Switching automatic processor rollers between developer and fixer.

         5) Using the same brush or sponge to clean developer and fixer automatic processor rollers or manual processing tanks.

      b. Corrective actions

         1) Use and maintain separate equipment for developer and fixer.

         2) Use care when handling processing chemistry. Cover tanks when not in use.

         3) Follow protocol for cleaning and maintaining manual processing film racks and other equipment.

         4) Label processing tanks and rollers to maintain separate developer and fixer contact.

         5) Label cleaning supplies for use with only the developer or with only the fixer.

I. Technique errors

  1. Resulting from incorrect image receptor placement (see Figures 4–20 and 4–21)

      a. Errors

         1) Too far anteriorly, posteriorly, superiorly, and inferiorly

         2) Not perpendicular to the embrasures and parallel to the facial surfaces of the teeth of interest

      b. Corrective actions

         1) Examine the patient's oral cavity for malaligned, missing, or supernumerary teeth, and adjust placement accordingly.

         2) Possess a working knowledge of which teeth must be imaged on each of the standard periapical and bitewing radiographs included in a full mouth survey.

  2. Resulting in horizontal overlap of the proximal surfaces of the teeth (see Figures 4–24 and 4–25)

      a. Errors

         1) Incorrect horizontal angulation of the x-ray beam

2) Incorrect placement of the image receptor perpendicular to the embrasures and parallel to the facial surfaces of the teeth of interest

   b. Corrective actions

      1) Align the x-ray beam to intersect the plane of the image receptor perpendicularly in the horizontal direction (see Figure 4–5).

      2) Determine whether the overlap is more severe in the anterior or the posterior region and then direct the PID so that the x-ray beam will strike slightly more from the anterior or from the posterior. Use the saying "Move toward it—the overlap—to fix it."

3. Resulting in incisal/occlusal edge or apices not recorded on the image (paralleling technique error)

   a. Errors

      1) Incorrect vertical angulation of the x-ray beam

      2) Incorrect positioning of the image receptor

   b. Corrective actions

      1) The x-ray beam must intersect the plane of the image receptor perpendicularly in the vertical dimension.

         a) Excessive vertical angulation results in not recording the incisal/occlusal edge (see Figure 4–22)

         b) Inadequate vertical angulation results in not recording the apices See Figure 4–23).

      2) Position the image receptor parallel to the teeth being imaged.

      3) Direct the patient to close down completely on the bite-block of the image receptor holder to ensure recording of the apices of the teeth of interest.

      4) Match the image receptor holding device with the technique used (paralleling device with the paralleling technique and bisecting device with the bisecting technique).

4. Resulting in elongation/foreshortening of the image (bisecting technique error)

   a. Errors

      1) Incorrect vertical angulation of the x-ray beam

      2) Incorrect positioning of the image receptor

      3) Film packet or PSP plate bending

         a) Patient applies too much pressure to image receptor while holding in place.

         b) Anatomical structures, such as tori, shallow palatal vault interfere with correct positioning.

   b. Corrective actions

      1) The x-ray beam must intersect the imaginary bisector between the plane of the image receptor and the long axis of the tooth perpendicularly in the vertical dimension.

         a) Excessive vertical angulation results in a foreshortened image (see Figure 5–20)

         b) Inadequate vertical angulation results in an elongated image (see Figure 5–21)

2) Place the image receptor as close to the teeth being imaged as possible without bending.

3) Inspect the oral cavity for possible obstructions and make adjustments as needed (see Laboratory Exercise 9, Patient Management and Student Partner Practice).

4) Direct the patient to close down completely on the bite-block of the image receptor holder to ensure recording of the apices of the teeth of interest.

5) Match the image receptor holding device with the technique used (paralleling device with the paralleling technique and bisecting device with the bisecting technique).

6) Do not use the patient's finger or thumb to hold the image receptor in place.

5. Resulting in a blurred image (poor resolution)

a. Errors

1) Movement of the patient, the image receptor, or the PID and tube head assembly

2) Slight enlargement that resembles blurring may occur when using a short (8-inch/20.5 cm) PID with greater image receptor-to-tooth distance used with the paralleling technique

b. Corrective actions

1) Establish good patient rapport to obtain maximum co-operation during the radiographic procedure. Educate the patient to the role they play in obtaining quality radiographs.

2) Ensure that the image receptor is correctly and securely positioned before making the exposure.

3) Do not use the patient's finger or thumb to hold the image receptor.

4) Ensure that the PID and tube head assembly are stable prior to exposure.

5) Replace a short 8-inch (20.5 cm) PID with one that is longer (12 inch/30 cm or 16 inch/41 cm).

REFERENCES

Carestream Health, Inc. (2007). *Kodak Dental Systems: Exposure and processing for dental film radiography.* Pub. N-414, Rochester, NY: Author.

Eastman Kodak Company. (2002). *Successful intraoral radiography.* N-418 CAT No. 103. Rochester, NY: Author.

Thomson, E. M., & Johnson, O. N. (2012). *Essentials of dental radiography for dental assistants and hygienists* (9th ed.). Upper Saddle River, NJ: Pearson.

White, S. C., & Pharoah, M. J. (2008). *Oral radiology principles and interpretation* (6th ed.). St. Louis, MO: Elsevier.

STUDY QUESTIONS

1. The ability to recognize errors made when taking dental radiographs will help the oral health care professional to:
   - A. Keep patient radiation exposure to a minimum.
   - B. Provide optimal oral health care for the patient.
   - C. Properly diagnose oral conditions.
   - D. Avoid retake radiographs.
   - E. All of the above

2. Each of the following is a characteristic of a quality periapical radiograph EXCEPT one. Which one is the EXCEPTION?
   - A. 2 mm of alveolar bone visible beyond the apex of each tooth
   - B. Density of the image not too light or too dark
   - C. Interproximal spaces appear overlapped
   - D. Image is an accurate representation of the teeth and supporting structures
   - E. Radiograph is free of technique and/or processing errors

3. Which of the following errors would result in a clear or blank radiograph?
   - A. No exposure to x-rays
   - B. Exposing the same image receptor twice
   - C. Extended developing time
   - D. Accidental white light exposure

4. Which of the following would result in herringbone error?
   - A. The film packet was bent prior to exposure.
   - B. The back of the film packet faced the x-ray beam during exposure.
   - C. The lead foil was chemically processed with the film.
   - D. The film was used to expose more than one area of the oral cavity.

5. After exposure to x-radiation, photostimuable phosphor (PSP) plates should be protected from bright light prior to scanning BECAUSE the PSP plate is erased by light exposure.
   - A. Both the statement and reason are correct and related.
   - B. Both the statement and reason are correct but NOT related.
   - C. The statement is correct, but the reason is NOT.
   - D. The statement is NOT correct, but the reason is correct.
   - E. NEITHER the statement NOR the reason is correct.

6. Radiographs that are too dark result from each of the following EXCEPT one. Which one is the EXCEPTION?
   - A. Developer solution was too hot.
   - B. Processing time was too long.
   - C. The developer chemical mix was overactive.
   - D. White light was leaking into the darkroom.
   - E. The film was placed in the fixer first.

7. The apices of the mandibular molar teeth in a periapical radiograph appear to be cut off the image. Which of the following errors is the most likely cause?

    A. Excessive horizontal angulation

    B. Inadequate horizontal angulation

    C. Excessive vertical angulation

    D. Inadequate vertical angulation

8. The image of the maxillary molar teeth in a periapical radiograph appears elongated. What should you do to improve this image?

    A. Decrease the horizontal angulation.

    B. Increase the horizontal angulation.

    C. Decrease the vertical angulation.

    D. Increase the vertical angulation.

9. Incorrect horizontal angulation results in which of the following errors?

    A. Conecutting

    B. Overlapping

    C. Reticulation

    D. Foreshortening

10. The overhead white light in the darkroom was turned on before a film was completely inserted into the automatic processor. This is the third time this month that this error has occurred. Describe the error created. Explain how and why the resulting image appears this way. What do you think is causing this error to occur so often? What corrective actions can you suggest to prevent this error from occurring?

_____

_____

_____

_____

_____

_____

_____

_____

_____

_____

laboratory exercise 8

Infection Control and Student Partner Practice

INTRODUCTION

The purpose of infection control is to prevent the transmission of disease between patients and between patients and oral healthcare providers. Cross-contamination through the creation of aerosols or through invasive procedures is not usually associated with radiographic procedures. However, infectious diseases may still be transmitted through saliva-contaminated radiographic equipment and supplies. Maintaining infection control throughout the radiographic process is particularly challenging. Keeping track of asepsis while moving in and out of the oral cavity can be challenging. Radiographic procedures further complicate the chain of asepsis by requiring movement in and out of the radiographic operatory itself. Furthermore, transporting contaminated image receptors to another location, such as the darkroom or to the location of the digital laser scanner, for further manipulation can make infection control a daunting responsibility. A thorough understanding of the recommended infection control protocols before, during, and after radiographic services is necessary to protect patients and oral healthcare providers from the transmission of disease. Additionally, the specific steps of these protocols require practice to achieve competency in skilled handling of contaminated radiographic equipment and supplies.

For this exercise, infection control protocols regarding oral radiography have been divided into four subcategories: (1) infection control prior, (2) during, and (3) after the radiographic procedure, and (4) infection control for the darkroom. While the fourth subcategory focuses on the processing procedure, the first three subcategories concentrate on the operatory where the radiographic procedure will be performed. The purpose of this exercise is to provide an opportunity to practice infection control protocols in these four subcategories. Through the use of role play, with a student partner, you will simulate exposing a series of bitewing radiographs on each other, establishing a real-life setting in which to practice infection control techniques.

OBJECTIVES

Following completion of this lab activity, you will be able to:

1. Demonstrate infection control protocol prior to, during, and after the radiographic procedure.

2. Demonstrate infection control protocol for the darkroom.

MATERIALS

Student partner

Lead/lead equivalent apron with thyroid collar

Size #2 radiographic film packets

Digital sensor and/or photostimuable phosphor (PSP) plates

Sterile or disposable bitewing image receptor holder for film, digital sensor, and/or PSP plate

Patient napkin/bib and chain

Handwashing station with antimicrobial soap or antiseptic hand rub

Disinfectant

Plastic or foil barriers

Paper towels

Disposable cups

Patient treatment gloves

Overgloves

Heavy duty utility gloves

Bitewing film mount

Tomato juice

PREPARATION

1. Study the chapter outline to prepare for this laboratory exercise. An understanding of the material presented in the outline is required to complete this activity.

2. Instructor demonstration may enhance knowledge of the laboratory exercise.

3. Select a student partner. Decide which student will play the role of the patient first and which student will play the role of the radiographer.

LABORATORY EXERCISE ACTIVITIES

Part 1: Exercise in Infection Control Protocol Prior to the Radiographic Procedure

1. Together with a student partner, prepare the radiographic operatory and obtain radiographic materials for this exercise. Follow the infection control guidelines prior to the radiographic procedure in Procedure

8–1. Use these guidelines to assess your ability to satisfactorily prepare the operatory for radiographic services.

2. Practice these infection control protocols until all steps can be performed at a mastery level.

Part 2: Exercise in Infection Control Protocol during the Radiographic Procedure

1. Before you begin Part 2 of this exercise, place a small amount, enough to completely coat four size #2 film packets, of tomato juice in the disposable paper cup. The tomato juice will simulate saliva contamination and will be used in Part 4 of this exercise.

2. With your student partner playing the role of the patient, proceed with the following steps:

   a. Inform patient of the need for radiographic services, explain procedure and rationale for radiographic services, answer patient concerns/questions regarding radiographic procedure, obtain patient's written consent for radiographic services.

   b. Seat patient.

   c. Request that the patient remove eyeglasses, removable dental appliances, and any other material that may interfere with the radiographic procedure such as chewing gum or facial jewelry adorning the nose, tongue, or lips.

   d. Adjust the height of the chair to a comfortable working level for the radiographer.

   e. Adjust the headrest so that the patient's midsagittal plane is perpendicular to the floor and the maxillary occlusal plane is parallel to the floor when imaging the maxilla and the mandibular occlusal plane is parallel to the floor when imaging the mandible.

   f. Place the lead/lead equivalent barrier with thyroid collar over the patient.

   g. Place a patient napkin/bib over the lead/lead equivalent apron (Figure 8–1 ■).

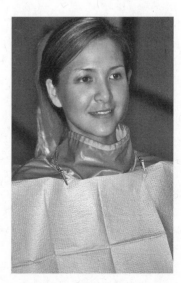

Figure 8–1 To aid in minimizing contamination, a patient napkin/bib may be placed over the lead/lead equivalent apron.

3. Place each film of the bitewing series intraorally. Position the x-ray tube head and PID for each projection. Follow the four basic steps of packet placement, vertical angulation, horizontal angulation, and centering the x-ray beam for exposing bitewing radiographs. (See Laboratory Exercise 2, Bitewing Radiographic Technique.)

   WARNING: DO NOT ACTIVATE THE EXPOSURE BUTTON. DO NOT EXPOSE YOUR STUDENT PARTNER TO RADIATION. YOU ARE PRACTICING PLACEMENT OF THE IMAGE RECEPTOR AND CORRECT X-RAY BEAM ALIGNMENT ONLY. YOU WILL NOT ACTUALLY EXPOSE THESE PRACTICE RADIOGRAPHS.

4. Follow the infection control guidelines during the radiographic procedure in Procedure 8–2. Use these guidelines to assess your ability to satisfactorily perform infection control during radiographic services. Practice these infection control protocols until all steps can be performed at a mastery level.

5. Obtain feedback on your image receptor placement, vertical and horizontal angulation, and centering of the x-ray beam as necessary or as directed by your instructor.

Part 3: Exercise in Infection Control Protocol after the Radiographic Procedure

1. When you have completed taking the simulated bitewing series of radiographs, follow the guidelines for infection control after the radiographic procedure in Procedure 8–3 to secure the radiography operatory.

Part 4: Exercise in Infection Control Protocol in the Darkroom

1. Transport the (simulated) exposed film packets to the darkroom or daylight loader processing area in the paper cup. Ensure that the films are completely coated with the tomato juice. In this exercise, the tomato juice is used to represent saliva contamination. In real life, excess saliva is removed from the image receptors by swiping each across a disinfectant-soaked paper towel immediately after removal from the oral cavity. While the tomato juice appears unrealistic, it does provide a visible indication of how well infection control protocols are being followed.

2. Process the films following the guidelines for infection control for the darkroom, Procedure 8–4. If your institution uses an automatic processor equipped with a daylight loader, choose Procedure 8–5.

3. Together with your student partner, use the darkroom assessment tool, Procedure 8–6, to evaluate your ability to follow the infection control protocols.

COMPETENCY AND EVALUATION

1. When the exercise is complete, discard films and materials and clean and disinfect the radiography operatory and the darkroom.

2. Switch student partner roles and repeat this exercise. The student "patient" should now play the role of radiographer, and the student radiographer should now play the role of "patient," so that both partners have the opportunity to complete this exercise.

3. Practice these infection control protocols until all steps can be performed at a mastery level.

4. Complete the study questions.

Procedure 8–1

Infection Control Prior to the Radiographic Procedure

Satisfactorily
Performed
✓

1. Put on PPE (personal protection equipment) barrier gown, eyewear, and mask. _____

2. Wash hands with an antimicrobial soap or use an antiseptic hand rub.* _____

3. Put on utility gloves.

4. Clean and disinfect with appropriate disinfectant all surfaces that will come in contact, either directly or indirectly, with the patient. See the following list:

   a. PID _____

   b. X-ray tube head _____

   c. Tube head support arms and handles _____

   d. Exposure button (push-button exposure switches may be damaged _____
   by the use of a disinfectant solution. Maintain infection control
   through the use of a plastic or foil barrier [Figure 8–2 ■]. Foot
   pedal exposure switches do not require disinfection.)

   e. Control panel dials (impulse timer, kVp, and mA controls) (control _____
   panel dials may be damaged by the use of a disinfectant solution.
   Maintain infection control through the use of a plastic or foil barrier
   [Figure 8–3 ■].)

   f. Patient chair including headrest, back support, armrests, body, _____
   and back of the chair

   g. Lead/lead equivalent apron/thyroid collar barrier _____

   h. Countertop and other work space areas _____

   i. Photostimuable phosphor (PSP) plates or digital sensors _____
   (as recommended by manufacturer)

5. Wash, dry, and remove utility gloves, and wash hands with an _____
   antimicrobial soap or use an antiseptic hand rub.

6. Put on clean overgloves. _____

(continued)

Procedure 8-1 (continued)

Satisfactorily
Performed
✓

7. Obtain plastic or foil barriers and cover all surfaces that will come in contact, either directly or indirectly, with the patient. See the following list:

   a. PID (Figure 8–4 ■)   _____

   b. X-ray tube head (Figure 8–4)   _____

   c. Tube head support arms and handles   _____

   d. Exposure button (Figure 8–2) (foot pedal exposure switches do not require a plastic or foil barrier.)   _____

   e. Control panel dials (impulse timer, kVp, and mA controls) procedure   _____

   f. Patient chair including headrest, back support, armrests, body, and back of the chair   _____

   g. Lead/lead equivalent apron/thyroid collar barrier (optional) (Figure 8–5 ■)   _____

   h. Countertop and other work space areas (Figure 8–6 ■)   _____

   i. Film packets (optional) (Figure 8–7 ■), PSP plates (see Figure 3–3), digital sensors (see Figure 3–2)   _____

8. Obtain radiographic supplies. See the following list:

   a. Film packets or PSP plates or digital sensor   _____

   b. Sterile or disposable image receptor holders   _____

   c. Film mount (for film-based radiography)   _____

   d. Disposable paper cup (for film packets) or containment box (for PSP plates) (Figure 8–8 ■ and see Figure 3–7)   _____

   e. Paper towels   _____

   f. Miscellaneous supplies (i.e., cotton rolls, extra disposable image receptor holders)   _____

9. Place the film mount under the plastic barrier on the counter work space (Figure 8–6).   _____

10. Place the film packets or PSP plates on the plastic barrier placed over the film mount (Figure 8–6).   _____

11. Saturate a folded paper towel with disinfectant and place next to the film mount on top of the plastic barrier (Figures 8–6 and 8–8).   _____

12. Prepare antimicrobial mouth rinse for patient use prior to procedure.**   _____

* When hands are visibly dirty, wash with an antimicrobial soap and water. If hands are not visibly soiled, an alcohol-containing preparation designed for reducing the number of viable microorganisms on the hands may be used. Refer to manufacturer's recommendations for use.

** Scientific evidence does not indicate that preprocedural mouth rinsing prevents the spread of infections; however, antimicrobial mouth rinses, for example, chlorhexidine gluconate, essential oils, or povidone-iodine, can reduce the number of microorganisms the patient might release in the form of aerosols or spatter during the radiographic procedure.

(continued)

Copyright © 2012 by Pearson Education, Inc.

Procedure 8-1 (continued)

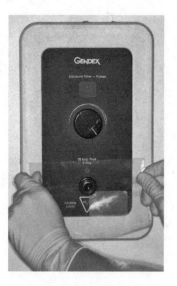

Figure 8–2 Use of a plastic barrier over the exposure button to maintain infection control.

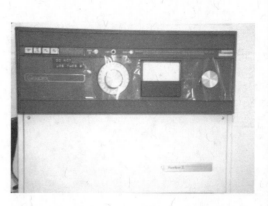

Figure 8–3 Use of adhesive-backed plastic barriers over the control panel dials to maintain infection control.

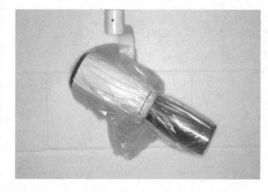

Figure 8–4 Use of plastic bag or plastic wrap over the x-ray tube head to maintain infection control.

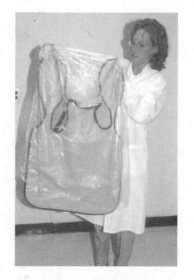

Figure 8–5 A plastic garment bag type barrier may be used to protect the lead/lead equivalent apron made of cloth or other material that can not be wiped with disinfectant.

(continued)

Procedure 8-1 (continued)

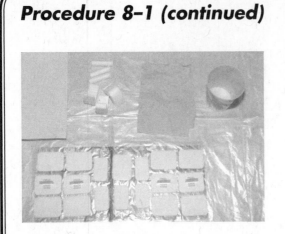

Figure 8–6 Countertop work space covered with plastic barrier and set up for exposure of a full mouth series of radiographs.

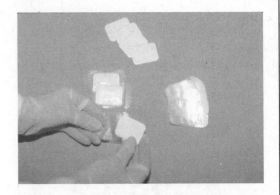

Figure 8–7 Commercially made plastic barrier envelopes may be placed over the film packet similar to barrier envelopes used to protect phosphor plates.

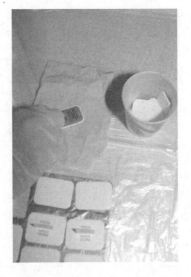

Figure 8–8 After exposure, the film is removed from the oral cavity and immediately swiped across a disinfectant-soaked paper towel to remove excess saliva.

Procedure 8-2

Infection Control during the Radiographic Procedure

1. After placing the lead/lead equivalent barrier with thyroid collar on the patient, remove overgloves, wash hands, and put on patient treatment gloves. _____

2. Assemble the image receptor into the appropriate holding device. Place intraorally and position the x-ray tube head and PID for each of the radiographs in the bitewing series. _____

3. Simulate exposure. _____

   WARNING: DO NOT EXPOSE YOUR STUDENT PARTNER TO RADIATION. REMEMBER THAT YOU ARE PRACTICING FILM PACKET PLACEMENT AND BEAM ALIGNMENT ONLY AND ARE NOT ACTUALLY EXPOSING THESE RADIOGRAPHS.

4. Film-based: Remove the image receptor and holder from patient's mouth following each exposure simulation, swipe across the disinfectant-saturated paper towel on the counter (Figure 8–8), and drop into the disposable paper cup receptacle. Do not touch the outside of the cup with contaminated treatment gloves. If covered with a plastic barrier envelope, locate the perforated edge and tear to open (Figure 8–9 ■). Allow the film to drop out into the cup without touching. _____

   PSP plates: Remove the image receptor and holder from patient's mouth following each exposure simulation and swipe across the disinfectant-saturated paper towel on the counter. Locate the perforated edge of the plastic barrier envelope and tear to open. Allow the plate to drop out into the containment box. Do not touch the plate or the containment box with contaminated treatment gloves.

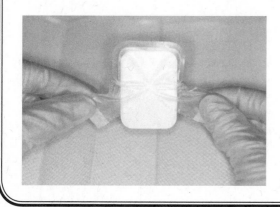

Figure 8–9 Aseptically opening a contaminated film packet sealed in a plastic barrier envelope.

(continued)

Procedure 8-2 (continued)

Digital sensor: Remove the image receptor and holder from patient's mouth following each exposure simulation. If necessary, use a paper towel to wipe excess saliva from the plastic barrier sheath. Do not remove the plastic barrier sheath until all exposures are completed.

5. Place and simulate exposure of all radiographs in this manner. _____

6. If additional supplies are needed that require contact with noncovered surfaces or the procedure must otherwise be interrupted, _____

   a. Rinse treatment gloves with plain water (no soap) and dry.*

   b. Place overgloves over treatment gloves.

   c. To restart the procedure, remove overgloves.

* If the procedure must be interrupted, the treatment gloves may be removed and discarded and the hands washed. Prior to restarting the procedure, the hands should be washed again and new treatment gloves put on.

Procedure 8-3

Infection Control after the Radiographic Procedure

Satisfactorily Performed ✓

1. Rinse, remove, and discard treatment gloves and wash hands with antimicrobial soap or use an antiseptic hand rub. _____

2. Remove lead/lead equivalent apron with thyroid collar barrier and dismiss patient. _____

3. Put on utility gloves. _____

4. PSP plates: Wipe with appropriate disinfectant (as recommended by manufacturer). _____

   Digital sensor: Remove plastic barrier sheath and discard. Wipe sensor with appropriate disinfectant (as recommended by manufacturer).

5. Prepare and package image receptor holders for sterilization according to manufacturer's directions. _____

6. Discard all disposable contaminated items such as disposable image receptor holders, paper towels, cotton rolls. _____

7. Remove and discard all plastic or foil barriers. _____

8. Clean and disinfect any uncovered surface. _____

9. Clean and disinfect lead/lead equivalent apron with thyroid collar barrier (if it was not covered with an impervious barrier). _____

10. Wash, dry, and remove utility gloves. _____

11. Wash hands with antimicrobial soap or use an antiseptic hand rub. _____

Procedure 8–4

Infection Control for the Darkroom

1. Obtain two paper towels. _____

2. Place one paper towel on the counter work space, and place the cup with contaminated films on this "contaminated" paper towel (Figure 8–10 ■). _____

3. Place the second paper towel on the counter work space, and keep this paper towel as the "uncontaminated" paper towel (Figure 8–10). _____

4. Secure darkroom door. _____

5. Turn off white overhead light and turn on safe light. _____

6. Put on a pair of clean treatment gloves. _____

7. Open each film packet (Figure 8–11 ■). _____

   a. Peel back the outer plastic/paper wrap using the tab on the back of the packet.

   b. Grasp the black paper with film sandwiched in between and pull straight out.

   c. Hold the black paper-film assembly over the designated uncontaminated paper towel and pull out slowly.

   d. Allow the film to drop out onto the paper towel. Do not touch the film with treatment gloves.

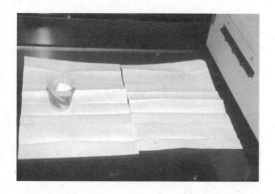

Figure 8–10 Darkroom counter work space with a contaminated area and an uncontaminated area. Note that this setup provides an orderly direction for the progression of darkroom activity. Contaminated film packets begin on the left. Packets are opened, and films are dropped into the uncontaminated area on the right, near the automatic processor loading area.

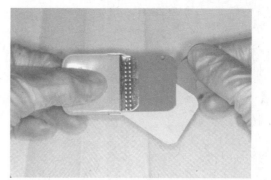

Figure 8–11 Aseptically opening a contaminated film packet.

(continued)

Procedure 8–4 (continued)

8. Drop the contaminated film packet outer plastic/paper wrap, black paper, and lead foil onto the "contaminated" paper towel. _____

9. Repeat steps 7 and 8 until all film packets have been opened (Figure 8–12 ■). _____

10. Rinse, remove, and discard treatment gloves and wash and dry hands. _____

11. With clean, dry hands, grasp by the edges and place films into the automatic processor feeder slots or load onto manual processing film racks and process following the manual processing procedure. _____

12. When all films have completely entered the automatic processing machine, or once the cover has been placed over the manual processing tanks, it is safe, turn on the overhead white light. _____

13. Put on heavy duty utility gloves and separate the lead foil from the film packets and discard as lead recycling waste. _____

14. Gather up contaminated paper towel with all waste and discard appropriately. _____

15. Clean and disinfect the counter work space. _____

16. Wash, dry, and remove utility gloves. _____

17. Wash and dry hands. _____

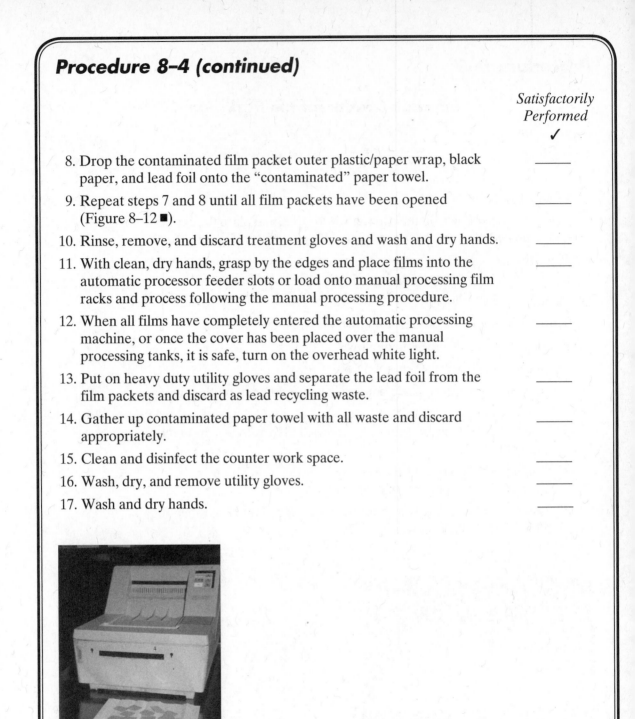

Figure 8–12 Illustration of the contaminated and uncontaminated areas when all film packets have been opened.

Procedure 8–5

Infection Control for Processors with Daylight Loaders

1. Obtain paper towels or plastic barrier sheet and new patient treatment gloves. _____

2. Open the light-filter cover and line the floor of the daylight loader compartment with a clean paper towel or plastic barrier. Designate a contaminated and an uncontaminated side of the floor of the compartment. _____

3. Place the cup with the film packets on the designated contaminated side, and a new pair of patient treatment gloves on the uncontaminated side inside the daylight loader compartment (Figure 8–13 ■). _____

4. Replace the light-filter cover. _____

5. Slide clean dry hands through the light-tight baffles.

6. Once inside, put on the pair of clean treatment gloves. _____

7. Open each film packet.

    a. Peel back the outer plastic/paper wrap using the tab on the back of the packet.

    b. Grasp the black paper with film sandwiched in between and pull straight out.

    c. Hold the black paper–film assembly over the designated uncontaminated side of the floor of the compartment and pull out slowly.

    d. Allow the film to drop out into the paper towel or plastic barrier. Do not touch the film with contaminated treatment gloves.

8. Drop the contaminated film packet onto the paper towel on the contaminated sided of the floor of the compartment. _____

9. Repeat steps 7 and 8 until all film packets have been opened. _____

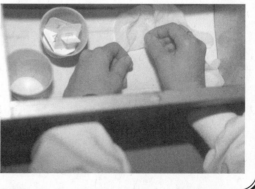

Figure 8–13 Daylight loader work space.

(continued)

Procedure 8–5 (continued)

10. Remove treatment gloves and place on the contaminated side of the paper towel on the floor of the compartment. _____

11. With clean, dry hands, grasp by the edges and place films into the automatic processor feeder slots for processing. _____

12. When the films are safely in the automatic processor, remove ungloved hands through the light-tight baffles. _____

13. Wash and dry hands. _____

14. Put on heavy duty utility gloves. _____

15. Open the light-filter cover, separate the lead foil from the film packets, and dispose of appropriately. Remove the cups, contaminated film packet outer plastic/paper wrap, and paper towels or plastic barrier and discard appropriately. _____

16. Clean and disinfect the inside of the compartment. _____

17. Wash, dry, and remove utility gloves. Disinfect.

18. Wash and dry hands. _____

Procedure 8-6

Darkroom Assessment Tool

Together with your partner, examine the following areas to assess your ability to maintain infection control in the darkroom during the film processing procedure. Place an (X) beside those areas where tomato juice was noted and an (O) beside those areas that remain uncontaminated.

Personal Space

__ Fingers/hands   __ Face/eyeglasses

__ Barrier gown/lab coat   __ Mask

Environment

__ Darkroom door   __ Paper towel dispenser

__ Light switches   __ Outside of processor

__ Walls   __ Outside of lead foil receptacle

__ Counter work space   __ Sink faucets

__ Pen/pencil holder   __ Other

I. Goals of infection control
   A. Prevent cross-contamination between patients
   B. Prevent cross-contamination between patient and radiographer
   C. Prevent cross-contamination between radiographer and other oral health care providers
II. Standard precautions
   A. Treat all body fluids (except sweat) as potentially infectious.
   B. Take precautions that prevent contact with all body fluids.
   C. Replaces the term universal precautions where the focus was on bloodborne pathogens.
III. Operator preparation
   A. Use of PPE (personal protective equipment)
      1. Impervious lab coat/barrier gown/scrubs
      2. Protective eyewear
      3. Mask
      4. Gloves
   B. Handwashing
      1. Remove rings, wristwatches, and other jewelry that can harbor microorganisms.
      2. Lather hands well with soap and rub vigorously for at least 15 seconds, or use an antiseptic hand rub following the manufacturer's directions for use.
IV. Classification of objects used in radiographic procedures
   A. Critical objects
      1. Objects that penetrate soft tissue or bone
      2. No critical objects are used in radiography
      3. Must be sterilized
   B. Semicritical
      1. Objects that contact but do not penetrate mucous membrane
      2. Image receptor holders, digital sensors, PSP plates
      3. Sterilized or disinfected with EPA-registered chemicals classified as high-level disinfectant. Digital sensors, PSP plates that cannot withstand sterilization must be wiped with a chemical disinfectant and covered with an impervious barrier prior to intraoral placement, then wiped again with chemical disinfectant after intraoral placement.
   C. Noncritical objects/clinical contact (environmental) surfaces
      1. Objects that contact the skin only and not the mucous membrane
      2. Objects that do not directly come into contact with the patient, but may be indirectly contaminated by contact from equipment used in the oral cavity or by contact by the contaminated gloved hands of the radiographer
      3. Lead/lead equivalent apron and thyroid collar and the countertops of the radiography operatory and darkroom
      4. Disinfected with EPA-registered chemicals classified as intermediate- or low-level disinfectant

V. Operatory preparation
   A. Clean and disinfect all surfaces that may be touched during the radiographic procedure.
   B. Spray-wipe-spray technique for most surfaces: Spray disinfectant on a paper towel and wipe switches and buttons that may otherwise be damaged by direct spray application.
   C. Cover with an impervious barrier all surfaces that can be covered, especially those that are difficult to disinfect.
   D. Use of impervious barriers help to reduce the amount of toxic disinfecting agents needed
   E. Examples of objects to be cleaned, disinfected, and covered:
      1. PID
      2. X-ray tube head (Figure 8–4)
      3. Tube head support arms and handles
      4. Exposure button (Figure 8–2)
      5. Control panel dials (Figure 8–3)
      6. Treatment chair including headrest, back support, armrests, body, and back of the chair
      7. Lead/lead equivalent apron/thyroid collar barrier that is made of cloth or other material that cannot be wiped with disinfectant (Figure 8–5)
      8. Countertop and other work space areas (Figure 8–6)
      9. Digital sensors and PSP plates
      10. Film packets (optional) (Figure 8–7)
   F. Supplies
      1. Use sterilized or disposable image receptor holders.
      2. Dispense image receptors from a central location.
         a. Obtain all image receptors required for the procedure at the same time.
         b. Use a clean disposable paper cup as the holding receptacle for transporting the image receptors.
         c. Image receptors may be prepackaged for ease in dispensing (Figure 8–14 ■).
      3. Plastic image receptor barrier envelopes and sheaths aid infection control
         a. Protect the film packet, PSP plate, and digital sensor from fluids in the oral cavity.
         b. The plastic barrier envelope should be opened immediately upon removing the film packet or PSP plate from the patient's oral cavity.

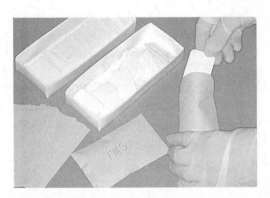

Figure 8–14 Film packets may be prepackaged for ease in dispensing.

1) Hold the image receptor over the cup (film) or containment box (PSP plate) and tear open the barrier envelope (Figure 8–9), allowing the image receptor to drop into the cup or containment box untouched by gloved hands.

2) Once all of the image receptors are exposed and opened in this manner, the cup will contain uncontaminated film packets that are ready to be transported to the darkroom for processing, and the box will contain uncontaminated PSP plates that are ready to be transported to the laser scanner location.

    c. The plastic barrier envelope protecting a wireless digital sensor or the barrier sheath protecting a wired digital sensor should remain in place until all exposures are completed.

G. Preparation of counter work space

    1. Place film packets and PSP plates to be exposed on a film mount that has been covered with a plastic barrier for ease in keeping track of exposures (Figure 8–6).

    2. Use a prepared disinfectant-soaked paper towel for removing excess saliva from the image receptors (Figure 8–8).

    3. Keep overgloves near the counter work space for easy placement over treatment gloves should the radiographic procedure be interrupted.

    4. Plan ahead; place extra disposable image receptor holders, paper towels, cotton rolls or other supplies out on the counter work space for easy access.

VI. Infection control during the radiographic procedure

A. Minimize area of contamination.

    1. Keep image receptors and holders confined to the prepared counter work space area when not in use.

    2. Remove excess saliva from image receptors immediately upon removing from the oral cavity.

    3. Minimize accidental saliva contamination of the lead/lead equivalent apron and thyroid collar through the use of a plastic barrier or patient napkin/bib (Figures 8–1 and 8–5).

B. Use overgloves if the radiographic procedure is interrupted.

    1. To attend to a matter outside of the immediate area

    2. To retrieve additional supplies during the procedure

    3. To touch an area not covered with a barrier

VII. Infection control after the radiographic procedure

A. Operatory and supplies

    1. Use heavy duty utility gloves for cleaning and disinfecting.

    2. Remove and discard all barriers.

    3. Clean and disinfect all surfaces that were not covered during the radiographic procedure.

    4. Prepare, package, and sterilize image receptor holding devices according to manufacturer's recommendations.

    5. Discard all disposable image receptor holding devices and other materials.

B. Transport exposed film packets to the area for processing and exposed PSP plates to the location of the laser scanner.

VIII. Infection control during the processing procedure
- A. Darkroom preparation
  1. Minimize area of contamination.
  2. Designate and prepare an area for contaminated materials.
  3. Assemble necessary supplies: paper towels, cups, pen/pencil, prior to opening the film packets.
- B. Procedure
  1. With treatment gloves on, pull up on the tab on the back of the film packet.
  2. Peel back the outer plastic/paper wrap.
  3. Grasp the black interleaf paper and pull straight out.
  4. Allow the film to drop onto a paper towel (Figure 8–11).
  5. Repeat until all film packets have been opened (Figure 8–12).
  6. Remove treatment gloves and wash and dry hands.
  7. Load films into the automatic processor or onto manual processing racks with clean, dry hands.
  8. Put on utility gloves.
  9. Discard contaminated materials appropriately.
  10. Clean and disinfect all surfaces that may have been touched during the procedure.
      a. Countertop work space
      b. Outside cabinet of the automatic processing unit
      c. Sink and faucets
      d. Overhead white light and safelight switches
      e. Pens/pencils
  11. Retrieve processed films with clean, dry hands.

REFERENCES

American Dental Association Council on Scientific Affairs. (2006). The use of dental radiographs: Update and recommendations. *J Am Dent Assoc, 137*(9), 1304–1312.

Darby, M. L., & Walsh, M. M. (2010). *Dental hygiene theory and practice* (3rd ed.). St. Louis, MO: Saunders Elsevier.

Dietz-Bourguignon, E., & Badavinac, R. (2002). *Safety standards and infection control for dental hygienists.* Albany, NY: Delmar, Thomson Learning.

Huber, M. A., Holton, R. H., & Terezhalmy, G. T. (2005). Cost analysis of hand hygiene using antimicrobial soap and water versus an alcohol-based hand rub. *Oral Surg Oral Med Oral Pathol, 99,* 4.

Infection Control in Practice, (2004, January) *3*(1). www.osap.org

Kalathingal, S. M., Moore, S., Kwon, S., Schuster, G. S., Shrout, M. K., & Plummer, K. (2009). An evaluation of microbiologic contamination on phosphor plates in a dental school. *Oral Surg Oral Med Oral Pathol, 107,* 279–282.

Kohn, W. G., Harte, J. A., Malvitz, D. M., Collins, A. S., Cleveland, J. L., & Eklund, K. J. (2004). Guidelines for infection control in dental health care settings—2003. *J Am Dent Assoc., 135,* 33–47.

Negron, W., Mauriello, S. M., Peterson, C. A., & Arnold, R. (2005). Cross-contamination of the PSP sensor in a preclinical setting. *J Dent Hyg, 79*(3), 1–10.

Organization for Safety and Asepsis Procedures: OSAP Check-Up: 2003 CDC Guidelines. (2004). Is your infection control program up to date? *Infection Control in Practice. Dentistry's Newsletter for Infection Control and Safety, 3*(1), 1–11.

Palenik, C. J. (2004). Infection control for dental radiography. *AADMRT Newsletter.* Retrieved December 13, 2010, from www.aadmrt.com/currents/palenik_fall_04_print.htm

Thomson, E. M., & Johnson, O. N. (2012). *Essentials of dental radiography for dental assistants and hygienists* (9th ed.). Upper Saddle River, NJ: Pearson.

U.S. Dept. of Health and Human Services for Disease Control and Prevention, Centers for Disease Control and Prevention. (2003, December 9). Guidelines for Infection Control in Dental Health-Care Settings. *MMWR* 52(RR17), 1–61.

U.S. Dept. of Health and Human Services for Disease Control and Prevention, Centers for Disease Control and Prevention. (2002, October 25). Guideline for Hand Hygiene in Health Care Settings: Recommendations of the Healthcare Infection Control Practices Advisory Committee and the HICPAC/SHEA/APIC/IDSA Hand Hygiene Task Force. *MMWR* 51(RR16), 1–44.

Wilkins, E. M. (2009). *Clinical practice of the dental hygienist* (10th ed.). Philadelphia: Lippincott Williams & Wilkins.

1. Each of the following is an example of PPE (personal protective equipment) EXCEPT one. Which one is the EXCEPTION?
   - A. Thyroid collar
   - B. Protective eyewear
   - C. Mask
   - D. Gloves

2. Which of these is classified as a semicritical object?
   - A. Tube head support arm
   - B. Image receptor holder
   - C. Lead/lead equivalent apron
   - D. Treatment chair

3. Each of the following must be disinfected prior to radiographic procedures EXCEPT one. Which one is the EXCEPTION?
   - A. X-ray machine tube head
   - B. Control panel
   - C. Film mount
   - D. Counter work space

4. Each of the following should be covered with an impervious barrier prior to radiographic procedures EXCEPT one. Which one is the EXCEPTION?
   - A. PID
   - B. Exposure switch
   - C. Treatment chair
   - D. Image receptor holding device

5. Which of the following would be indicated for the operator during the radiographic procedure?
   - A. Barrier gown, patient treatment gloves
   - B. Barrier gown, patient treatment gloves, protective eyewear
   - C. Barrier gown, patient treatment gloves, mask
   - D. Barrier gown, patient treatment gloves, protective eyewear, mask

6. Which of the following describes the purpose of wiping the image receptor with a disinfectant-soaked paper towel following exposure?
   - A. To eliminate the need for a containment box
   - B. To remove excess saliva
   - C. To eliminate the need for gloves during processing
   - D. To meet regulations for handling a biohazard

7. Which of the following should be used when opening film packets without plastic barrier envelopes?
   - A. Treatment gloves
   - B. Overgloves
   - C. Heavy duty utility gloves
   - D. Clean, dry hands

8. Once films have been separated from the contaminated outer plastic/paper wrap, black paper, and lead foil, films should be loaded into the processor with
    A. Treatment gloves
    B. Overgloves
    C. Heavy duty utility gloves
    D. Clean, dry hands

9. Which of the following infection control methods is required for intraoral digital sensors?
    A. Wash with soap and water and cover with a plastic barrier.
    B. Ultrasonic with detergent and dry heat sterilize.
    C. Disinfect and cover with a plastic barrier.
    D. Disinfect and autoclave (moist heat under pressure).
    E. Wash with soap and water, ultrasonic with detergent, autoclave sterilize, and then cover with a plastic barrier just prior to use.

10. While attempting to place an intraoral film packet into the oral cavity of the patient, you accidentally drop the film packet on the floor. In the space below, indicate how you would maintain infection control in this situation. List specific steps you would take in responding to this dilemma.

_____

_____

_____

_____

_____

_____

_____

_____

_____

_____

_____

_____

Patient Management and Student Partner Practice

INTRODUCTION

Ideal image receptor placement may not be easily achieved on all patients. In radiography, as in other areas of oral health care, each patient presents a unique situation. Although it is important to understand and become proficient in the theory and basic skills required to perform radiographic procedures, the radiographer must be prepared to modify basic techniques. Having a working knowledge of acceptable deviations from the basic techniques that do not compromise radiographic quality are skills of an outstanding radiographer. The ability to overcome predictable obstacles to achieving ideal image techniques should be part of the radiographer's repertoire.

The purpose of this laboratory exercise is twofold. First, this exercise facilitates the transfer of the skills you have mastered on teaching manikins or skulls to the clinical setting with a real patient or a student partner. Second, through the use of role-play, student partners provide critical feedback not only to improve radiographic technique skills, but also for development of patient management skills.

OBJECTIVES

Following completion of this lab activity, you will be able to:

1. Demonstrate proficiency in placing intraoral image receptors and aligning the vertical and horizontal angulation and centering the x-ray beam.

2. Maintain an organized and orderly work space area that is conducive to a systematic flow of the radiographic procedure.

3. Determine when to use the bisecting technique.

4. Adapt basic radiographic techniques to obtain quality diagnostic images when presented with a patient
   a. Who is apprehensive
   b. With a hypersensitive gag reflex

c. With a large palatal/mandibular tori/shallow palate

d. With a tight lingual frenulum/large muscular tongue

5. Knowledgeably and confidently respond to patient questions and concerns regarding the radiographic procedure.

MATERIALS

Size #1 and size #2 radiographic films, photostimuable phosphor (PSP) plates, or digital sensors

Sterile or disposable bitewing and periapical image receptor holders

Student partner

Lead/lead equivalent barrier with thyroid collar

Patient napkin/bib and chain

Handwashing station with antimicrobial soap or antiseptic hand rub

Disinfectant

Plastic or foil barriers

Paper towels

Disposable cups

Patient treatment gloves

Disposable overgloves

Heavy duty utility gloves

Full mouth series film mount

PREPARATION

1. Study the chapter outline to prepare for this laboratory exercise. An understanding of the material presented in the outline is required to complete this activity.

2. Instructor demonstration may enhance knowledge of the laboratory exercise.

3. Select a student partner. Decide which student will play the role of the patient first and which student will play the role of the radiographer.

4. Then switch student partner roles and repeat this exercise so that both partners have the opportunity to complete this exercise as the radiographer and as the patient.

LABORATORY EXERCISE ACTIVITIES

Part 1: Exercise in the Radiographic Procedure

1. Together with a student partner, prepare the radiographic operatory and obtain radiographic materials for this exercise. Follow infection control

guidelines for setting up the operatory. (See Laboratory Exercise 8, Infection Control and Student Partner Practice, Procedure 8–1.)

2. With your student partner playing the role of the patient, proceed with the following steps:

    a. Inform patient of the need for radiographic services, explain procedure and rationale for radiographic services, answer concerns/questions regarding radiographic procedure, obtain patient's written consent for radiographic services.

    b. Seat the patient.

    c. Request that the patient remove eyeglasses, removable dental appliances, and any other material that may interfere with the radiographic procedure, such as chewing gum or facial jewelry adorning the nose, tongue, or lip.

    d. Adjust the height of the chair to a comfortable working level for the operator.

    e. Adjust headrest so that the patient's midsagittal plane is perpendicular to the floor and maxillary occlusal plane is parallel to the floor when imaging the maxilla and the mandibular occlusal plane is parallel to the floor when imaging the mandible.

    f. Place the lead/lead equivalent apron with thyroid collar over the patient.

    g. Place a patient napkin/bib over the lead/lead equivalent apron.

3. Refer to the guidelines for infection control during the radiographic procedure outlined in Procedure 8–2. (See Laboratory Exercise 8, Infection Control and Student Partner Practice.) You may perform this exercise using film, photostimuable phosphor (PSP) plates, or a digital sensor. The size and/or number of radiographs that make up a full mouth series varies among practices. Refer to the various configurations illustrated in Figure 4–3 (see Laboratory Exercise 4, Periapical Radiographs—Paralleling Technique) to determine the number and size of image receptors you will need. This exercise will use the full mouth series configuration shown in Figure 4.3A. Place the image receptor into position intraorally. Then position the x-ray tube head and PID for each projection. If you are practicing the paralleling technique, direct the vertical angulation perpendicular to the plane of the image receptor and the long axis of the tooth. If you are practicing the bisecting technique, direct the vertical angulation perpendicular to the imaginary bisector between the plane of the image receptor and the long axis of the tooth. Follow the basic four steps of image receptor placement, vertical angulation, horizontal angulation, and centering the x-ray beam.

WARNING: DO NOT ACTIVATE THE EXPOSURE BUTTON. DO NOT EXPOSE YOUR STUDENT PARTNER TO RADIATION. YOU ARE PRACTICING PLACEMENT OF THE IMAGE RECEPTOR AND CORRECT X-RAY BEAM ALIGNMENT ONLY. YOU WILL NOT ACTUALLY EXPOSE THESE PRACTICE RADIOGRAPHS.

4. When you have positioned the image receptor and have aligned the x-ray tube head and PID, have your instructor evaluate your performance and record your progress, using the *Instructor Evaluation and Feedback Form* that follows. Do not wait after each radiograph is placed for your instructor to initial each projection; instead, continue practicing placement, vertical and horizontal angulation, and centering of the x-ray beam. Obtain feedback as necessary or as directed by your instructor.

Part 2: Role-play in Special Patient Management

1. When acting in the role of student partner patient, assume each one of the following patient roles:
   a. An apprehensive patient
   b. A patient with a hypersensitive gag reflex
   c. A patient with large palatal and/or mandibular tori and/or shallow palate
   d. A patient with a tight lingual frenulum and/or large muscular tongue

   The questions and comments that accompany each of the roles will guide you in acting realistically to challenge your partner to adapt basic radiographic techniques to achieve the goal of producing diagnostic quality radiographs.

2. Throughout the role-play, provide feedback for your partner, both on procedures done well and on those areas in need of improvement.

COMPETENCY AND EVALUATION

1. When the exercise is complete, discard the films and materials appropriately. The practice films were not actually exposed and will not be processed.

2. Follow infection control guidelines for the radiographic procedure outlined in Procedure 8–3. (See Laboratory Exercise 8, Infection Control and Student Partner Practice.)

3. When both you and your partner have completed the exercise, each of you should reflect on the experience of being the patient and write out your answers to the questions listed on the Instructor Evaluation and Feedback form that follows.

4. Complete the study questions.

NAME _____

INSTRUCTOR EVALUATION AND FEEDBACK FORM

Projection	Instructor's Initials
Right maxillary canine periapical	_____
Maxillary central incisors periapical	_____
Left maxillary canine periapical	_____
Left mandibular canine periapical	_____
Mandibular central incisors periapical	_____
Right mandibular canine periapical	_____
Right maxillary premolar periapical	_____
Right maxillary molar periapical	_____
Right mandibular premolar periapical	_____
Right mandibular molar periapical	_____
Right premolar bitewing	_____
Right molar bitewing	_____
Left maxillary premolar periapical	_____
Left maxillary molar periapical	_____
Left mandibular premolar periapical	_____
Left mandibular molar periapical	_____
Left premolar bitewing	_____
Left molar bitewing	_____

STUDENT PARTNER EVALUATION

What strengths did your partner demonstrate as the radiographer?

Why do you consider these strengths?

What specific actions would you suggest for improvement?

How was your partner's chairside manner?

What did he or she say to put you at ease with the procedure?

What could have been done better?

Were your questions/concerns regarding the procedure appropriately addressed?

What did your partner say or do to encourage your cooperation with the procedure?

Did you notice other actions during the procedure such as infection control, handling of equipment, attire of your partner, and so on?

What were your thoughts while you were the patient?

Can you imagine your future patients having these same thoughts?

Will they be positive? If not, what can you do to help increase the likelihood of a positive experience for your future patients?

Procedure 9–1

Special Patients Role-Play and Suggested Dialogue

Apprehensive Patient

This patient may be embarrassed by nervous feelings and may not tell you verbally that he or she is apprehensive. Instead, body language, talking rapidly or not at all, and an anxious demeanor may be observed. This patient may have had unpleasant past experiences that make him or her fearful. Nervousness may sometimes prompt the apprehensive patient to assume a defensive attitude and become angry if the procedure is not completed quickly. This may occur as the patient's stress level builds during the procedure. Sample dialogue for role-playing the apprehensive patient:

"Is this going to hurt?"

"How long is this going to take?"

"Are you trained to do this?"

"Why isn't the dentist doing this herself?"

"Last time the dentist told me I didn't need all of these. Why do I need all of them now?"

Hypersensitive Gag Reflex

This patient may talk about gagging prior to the procedure or may not bring it up until it occurs. The patient may be embarrassed by this reaction and may get upset that he or she cannot control this urge. This patient may have had an unpleasant experience with gagging in the past and may be nervous that it will be repeated now. Some patients may actually announce proudly that he or she is the biggest gagger you've ever encountered. Sample dialogue for role-playing the patient with a hypersensitive gag reflex:

"I'm a gagger,"

"Last time I had x-rays I gagged."

"Will these x-rays cause me to gag?"

"Can you do something so I won't gag during this procedure?"

"Last time, the dental hygienist let me try to put the holder in my own mouth. Can I try?"

Large Palatal or Mandibular Tori/Shallow Palate

Patients with tori do not usually present a problem for radiographic procedures. It is when the torus is large and/or when combined with a shallow palatal vault that placement of the image receptor becomes difficult. Large tori prevent alignment of the image receptor parallel with the long axis of the tooth and can make it difficult to position the image receptor far enough anteriorly to image the canine and first premolar. Mandibular tori may be so large as to extend across the floor of the mouth, making it impossible to place

(continued)

Procedure 9–1 (continued)

the receptor into the sublingual area. An additional concern is that the mucosa covering the torus is often sensitive to stimulation. Use this patient role-play situation to practice the bisecting technique. Sample dialogue for role-playing the patient with large palatal or mandibular tori or a shallow palate:

"I can't close down."

"Something is hitting the roof of my mouth."

"It feels like something is cutting the floor of my mouth."

"Last time the dental hygienist bent the film or something. Will you do this?"

Tight Lingual Frenulum/Large Muscular Tongue

The patient with a tight lingual frenulum or large muscular tongue may make placement of mandibular periapical and bitewing radiographs difficult. The "tongue-tied" patient may complain of sensitive mucosa, especially if the image receptor scrapes across this area. A muscular tongue and a tensing of the muscles in the sublingual area can interfere with image receptor placement by blocking access to the sublingual area. Use this patient role-play situation to practice the bisecting technique. Sample dialogue for role-playing the patient with a tight lingual frenulum or large muscular tongue:

"My tongue seems to be in the way."

"Where do you want me to position my tongue?"

"It feels like the holder is too big for my mouth."

"Can you place the film on top of my tongue?"

I. Special patient management
   A. Be prepared to adapt basic techniques.
   B. Recognize situations that call for adaptation of basic techniques.
   C. Possess a repertoire of acceptable variations of ideal techniques.
   D. Maintain confidence and authority throughout the radiographic procedure.
   E. Be firm yet gentle in instruction to the patient.

II. Apprehensive patient
   A. Causes
      1. Often consider the radiographic procedure to be unpleasant
      2. Unpleasant past experience may contribute to anxiety level
      3. May become apprehensive if the radiographer projects negativity or lack of confidence
   B. Prevention
      1. Develop a rapport that demonstrates attentive listening and empathy.
      2. Maintain confidence and authority.
      3. Reassure the patient and show appreciation for his or her cooperation with the procedure.

III. Patient with a hypersensitive gag reflex
   A. Causes
      1. Psychogenic stimuli—originating in the mind
         a. May be stimulated by the suggestion of a gag reflex
         b. Past experience with a gag reflex may predispose future episodes
      2. Tactile stimuli—resulting from physical touch
         a. Reaction to stimulus blocking the airway
         b. Low tolerance to foreign objects in the oral cavity
   B. Prevention
      1. Maintain confidence and authority throughout the radiographic procedure.
      2. Do not suggest a gagging response if the patient does not bring it up.
      3. If the patient initiates discussion of the gag reflex, allow ample time to communicate concerns; use listening skills to gain the patient's confidence; do not dismiss patient's concerns; empathize.
      4. Explain the radiographic procedure and your prevention techniques to gain the patient's confidence.
      5. Encourage patient's questions regarding the procedure and be prepared to give direct and frank answers to the patient's concerns.
      6. Begin the radiographic procedure by placing the image receptor into those positions least likely to excite a gag reflex; for most patients this would mean beginning in the anterior region.
      7. Do not slide the edge of the film packet or seam edge of the plastic barrier envelope on the PSP plate or sheath on the digital sensor across sensitive mucosa as this may feel sharp to the patient; instead, try to place directly into position.

8. Prepare for the exposure prior to placement of the image receptor by setting the exposure factors, estimating the vertical and horizontal angulation, and then place and expose the radiograph quickly.

9. Demonstrate placement of the image receptor intraorally prior to actual placement by using a finger to massage the tissue.

C. Suppressing once initiated

1. Begin the procedure over again, utilizing one of the above prevention techniques or the bisecting technique.

2. Use a distraction technique.

   a. Use an image receptor holder that the patient can be encouraged to clench teeth and bite down on.

   b. Direct concentration to another part of the body during the procedure.

      1) Raise a leg/arm.

      2) Wiggle a finger (Figure 9–1 ■).

      3) Press the back of the head against the headrest.

   c. Employ breathing exercises.

      1) Request that patient hold breath during the exposure.

      2) Request that patient concentrate on taking a number of slow deep breaths during the exposure.

      3) Request that the patient hum throughout the exposure, first explaining that the gag reflex may be initiated by the body's illusion of not being able to breathe.

3. Individualize treatment

   a. Before trying any method, whether scientific or gimmick, for suppressing the gag reflex, explain the technique to the patient, allow the power of suggestion of individualized treatment to assist in suppressing the gag reflex.

      1) Use a smaller-sized image receptor.

      2) Switch to a different image receptor holder.

      3) Apply a product such as cushion to the edge of the image receptor (Figures 9–2 ■ and 9–3 ■).

   b. Use stimulation of the senses of taste and feeling to "confuse" the gag reflex.

      1) Request that the patient rinse with an antiseptic mouth rinse or cold water just prior to placing the image receptor.

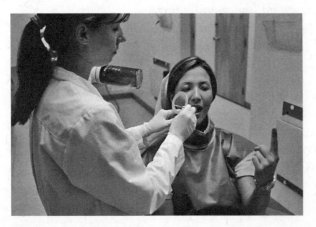

Figure 9–1 Patient attention is directed to another part of the body during the procedure.

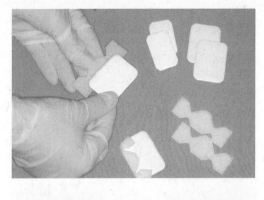

Figure 9–2 Applying a commercially made edge protector to a film packet.

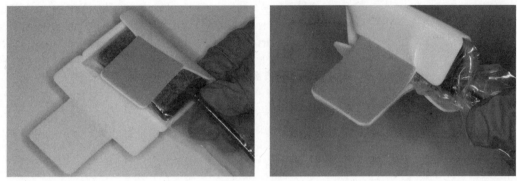

Figure 9–3 Commercially made edge protector with bite tab applied to a digital sensor.

      2) Use a film packet that has just been removed from cold refrigerator storage.

      3) Apply a small amount of table salt to the middle or the tip of the tongue just prior to placing the image receptor.

    c. Do not begin the radiographic procedure using any of the above. Instead "save" these techniques to introduce in conjunction with the power of suggestion. (For some patients, especially those who seem proud of the fact that they are the "best gaggers in the world," it may be best to allow for the stimulation of the gag reflex first before trying one of the above methods. Some individuals need to prove that they are gaggers and then will be responsive to suggestions for suppression.)

  D. Severe gag reflex

    1. Dentist may prescribe a topical anesthesia.

      a. Introducing a medical agent brings risks.

      b. A numbing sensation, especially in the soft palate and oral pharyngeal area, may cause some patients anxiety and could worsen the gag reflex.

    2. An extra oral radiographic procedure may have to be employed.

IV. Large torus palatinus (maxillary) or torus mandibularis (mandibular) (plural = tori)

  A. Problems encountered during radiographic procedures

    1. Radiographer may not be able to place the image receptor accurately in relation to the teeth in the region of the torus.

    2. Film packet and PSP plate may bend during placement.

3. Patient may not be able to bite down all the way on the image receptor holding device (Figure 9–4 ■).
4. Placing the image receptor on top of the palatal tori may result in the apices of the maxillary teeth not being recorded (Figure 9–4).
5. Mandibular tori may be large enough to extend all the way across the sublingual area, prohibiting image receptor placement.
6. Mandibular tori increase the chance that image receptor placement may be uncomfortable.
7. Large, dense tori appear radiopaque on the resulting image and may obscure diagnostic information.

B. Solutions
1. When placing the image receptor to expose maxillary periapical radiographs, use the midline where the palatal vault is the highest.
2. If the torus is large enough to interfere with image receptor placement, place the image receptor behind the torus (Figures 9–5 ■ and 9–6 ■).

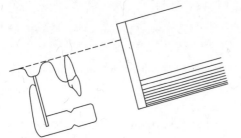

Figure 9–4 Resting the image receptor on top of a large palatal torus may prevent the patient from occluding on the biteblock of the holder. Note that the apices of the teeth will not be recorded.

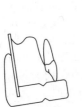
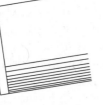
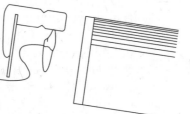

Maxillary film placement

Mandibular film placement

Figure 9–5 The image receptor should be placed behind large tori to maintain a parallel relationship between the long axis of the tooth and the plane of the image receptor.

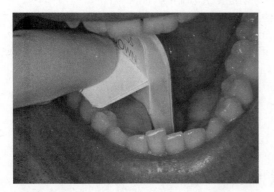

Figure 9–6 Placing the image receptor behind the torus maintains a parallel relationship between the long axes of the teeth and the plane of the image receptor.

3. When placing the image receptor to expose mandibular periapical radiographs, place a finger on the sensitive mucosa over the tori to protect it while positioning the image receptor intraorally.

4. Apply an edge protector to the image receptor (Figures 9–2 and 9–3).

5. When the tori cause image receptor placement to be only slightly off from parallel to the long axis of the tooth, a diagnostic image is still achievable by increasing the vertical angulation 5 to 15 degrees (Figure 9–7 ■).

6. When the tori cause image receptor placement to be more than 5 to 15 degrees off from parallel to the long axis of the tooth, use the bisecting technique and increase the vertical angulation to compensate for the flatter position of the image receptor.

7. Large, dense tori may require an increase in kilovoltage (kVp) to allow the x-ray beam to penetrate the structure.

V. Shallow palatal vault
   A. Problems encountered during radiographic procedures
      1. Placement of the image receptor parallel to the tooth may not be possible.
      2. Film packet and PSP plate may bend during placement.
      3. Patient may not be able to bite down all the way on the image receptor holding device.
      4. If the palate is also narrow, the image receptor may become wedged between the left and right alveolar ridges.
   B. Solutions
      1. Use a smaller-sized image receptor with a 5 to 15 degree increase in vertical angulation.
      2. Substitute a smaller, lightweight image receptor holding device.
      3. When the palate causes image receptor placement to be only slightly off from parallel to the long axis of the tooth, a diagnostic image is still achievable by increasing the vertical angulation 5 to 15 degrees.
      4. When the palate causes image receptor placement to be more than 5 to 15 degrees off from parallel to the long axis of the tooth, utilize the bisecting technique.

VI. Tight lingual frenulum/large, muscular tongue
   A. Problems encountered during radiographic procedures
      1. Film packet and PSP plate may bend during placement.
      2. Muscular tongue may prevent access to the sublingual area.

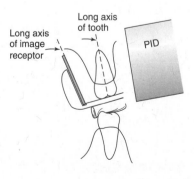

Figure 9–7 When the lack of parallelism is less than 15 degrees, the resultant image will generally be acceptable. The radiographer may choose to increase the vertical angulation 5 to 15 degrees to compensate for this lack of parallelism.

3. Lack of tongue control or an involuntary reaction may prompt the tongue to try to push the image receptor out of the mouth.
4. If an attempt is made to rest the image receptor on top of the tongue, the patient may not be able to bite down all the way on the holder (Figure 9–8 ■).
5. Placing the image receptor on top of the tongue may result in image receptor movement and/or not recording the apices of the mandibular teeth (Figure 9–8).
6. Restrictive tongue movement may require sliding the image receptor into place, increasing the sensation of scraping sensitive mucosa.
7. Tight sublingual musculature may prohibit placement of the image receptor parallel to the long axis of the tooth.

B. Solutions
1. Massage the sublingual area to help relax the tight sublingual musculature and acclimate the tongue to the position of the image receptor.
2. When placing the image receptor, place a finger on the sensitive mucosa over the alveolar ridge to protect it while positioning the image receptor intraorally.
3. Before initial placement of the image receptor, request that the patient close halfway to relax the tight frenulum and sublingual musculature; as the patient closes the rest of the way, ease the image receptor into place.

VII. Edentulous areas
A. Problems encountered during radiographic procedures
1. Lack of tooth/teeth to stabilize image receptor holding device.
2. Image receptor holder may tip into the edentulous space.
3. No long axis of the tooth to align the image receptor parallel to.
4. Lack of density in the edentulous area may cause an increased radiolucency that may mimic pathosis on the resulting image.

B. Solutions
1. Experiment with different image receptor holding devices.
2. Use cotton rolls or rolled 2 × 2 gauze squares to "fill" in an edentulous area.
3. If sufficient alveolar ridge remains intact in the edentulous area, two cotton rolls can be attached to the image receptor holding device to maintain a parallel relationship between image receptor and alveolar ridge (Figure 9–9 ■).
4. Estimate the long axis of the alveolar ridge to determine the correct vertical angulation.

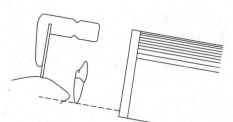

Figure 9–8 Resting the image receptor on top of the tongue may prevent the patient from occluding on the biteblock of the holder. Note that the apices of the teeth will not be recorded.

5. When a parallel relationship between the long axis of the edentulous ridge and the image receptor is not possible, utilize the bisecting technique.

6. Completely edentulous areas are less dense, and therefore require 25 percent less radiation exposure than those areas with teeth present.

VIII. Malaligned teeth

  A. Problems encountered during radiographic procedures

    1. Horizontal overlap

    2. Not recording all the appropriate teeth on one radiograph

  B. Solutions

    1. Increase the number of image receptors exposed.

    2. Use two different horizontal angles to overcome overlapping error.

      a. Examine the area of malaligned teeth and note the different horizontal angulations needed to complete the survey (Figure 9–10 ■).

      b. Align the horizontal angulation for the standard exposure and obtain the first exposure.

      c. Expose a second radiograph, aligning the horizontal angulation such that the x-ray beam will be directed perpendicularly through the contact area of the malaligned teeth.

      d. When altering the horizontal angulation to expose a malaligned area, the image receptor position should also be altered such that the x-ray beam will intersect it perpendicularly.

IX. Radiographic procedures for the child patient

  A. Considerations

    1. Smaller oral cavity

    2. Shallow palatal vault

    3. Shallow sublingual area

    4. Fear of unknown procedure

    5. Cooperation levels may vary

    6. Lack of tongue, muscle control

    7. Exfoliating and erupting teeth may lead to increased mucosa sensitivity

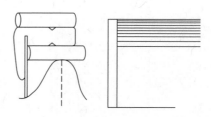

Figure 9–9 If there is sufficient alveolar ridge remaining in an edentulous area, two cotton rolls will aid in placing the image receptor parallel to the long axis of the edentulous ridge.

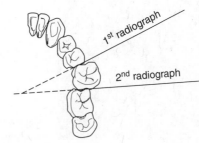

Figure 9–10 Two radiographs, using two different horizontal angulations, may be required to accurately image an area with malaligned teeth.

B. Determining the size and number of radiographs depends on:
1. Oral health care needs
2. Age of the patient and teeth erupted
3. Size of the mouth opening and oral cavity
4. Sensitivity of the oral mucosa
5. Child's attention span and ability to understand instructions and cooperate with the procedure
C. Management
1. Utilize a "show-tell-do" approach to gain the patient's confidence.
2. Explain the radiographic procedure and what is expected of the patient in understandable terms.
3. Use smaller image receptor sizes.
4. Modify the image receptor holding device for patient comfort and manageability (Figure 9–11 ■).
5. When a parallel relationship between the long axis of the tooth and the image receptor is not possible, utilize the bisecting technique.
6. When image receptor placement is difficult, an occlusal technique may be employed (Figure 9–12 ■). (See Exercise 10, Occlusal Radiographic Technique.)
7. When cooperation is difficult, employ caregiver's assistance. Provide the caregiver with the appropriate lead/lead equivalent barriers if he or she will be in the path of the primary beam during exposure.

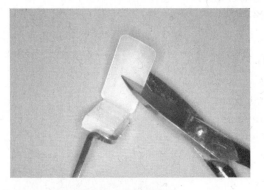

Figure 9–11 Modifying an image receptor holding device to adapt to a child's smaller oral cavity.

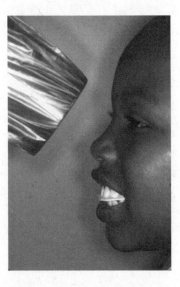

Figure 9–12 Placement of the image receptor for use with the occlusal technique is usually well tolerated by the child patient.

D. Exposure settings for children
   1. Children under age 10—reduce exposure settings to half those used for exposure of adult radiographs.
   2. Children age 10 to 15—reduce exposure settings by one-third of those used for exposure of adult radiographs.
   3. Children over age 15—exposure settings are the same as those used for adult radiographs.
E. Recommended image receptor size and number
   1. Primary dentition
      a. Prior to the eruption of the first permanent tooth (approximately 3 to 6 years of age)
      b. Bitewing examination—two posterior image receptor size #0 or #1
      c. Full mouth examination—one maxillary and one mandibular occlusal image receptor size #2
   2. Transitional (mixed primary and permanent) dentition
      a. Following the eruption of the first permanent tooth and prior to the eruption of the second permanent molars (approximately 7 to 12 years of age)
         1) Bitewing examination—two posterior image receptor size #1 or #2
         2) Full mouth examination—ten periapical radiographs (three maxillary anterior, three mandibular anterior, one posterior in all four quadrants) image receptor size #1 or #2
      b. Following the eruption of the second permanent molars (after age 12), utilize the same bitewing and full mouth series of radiographs as used for adult patients
         1) Bitewing examination—four posterior image receptor size #2
         2) Full mouth examination—fourteen periapicals (three maxillary anterior, three mandibular anterior, two posterior in all four quadrants), image receptor size #2 for all, or a combination of image receptor size #2 in the posterior regions and image receptor size #1 in the anterior regions

REFERENCES

Eastman Kodak Company (2002). *Successful intraoral radiography*. N-418 CAT No. 103, Rochester, NY: Author.

Pinkham, J. R., Casamassimo, P. S., Fields, H. W., McTigue, D. J., & Nowak, A. J. (2005). *Pediatric dentistry infancy through adolescence* (4th ed.). St. Louis, MO: Elsevier Saunders.

Thomson, E. M. (1993). Dental radiographs for the child patient. *Dent Hyg News*, 6, 19–20, 24.

Thomson, E. M. & Johnson, O. N. (2012). *Essentials of dental radiography for dental assistants and hygienists* (9th ed.). Upper Saddle River, NJ: Pearson.

White, S. C., & Pharoah, M. J. (2008). *Oral radiology principles and interpretation* (6th ed.). St. Louis, MO: Elsevier.

Wilkins, E. M. (2010). *Clinical practice of the dental hygienist* (10th ed.). Philadelphia: Lippincott Williams & Wilkins.

1. Which of the following projections is most likely to initiate a gag reflex?

    A. Premolar bitewing radiograph
    B. Molar bitewing radiograph
    C. Mandibular canine periapical radiograph
    D. Maxillary molar periapical radiograph

2. Which of the following would be the best method for preventing a gag reflex?

    A. Apply a topical anesthetic.
    B. Use salt on the tip of the tongue.
    C. Provide instruction confidently.
    D. Rinse with an antiseptic mouth rinse.

3. Each of the following is considered an appropriate distraction technique to help the patient cope with a hypersensitive gag reflex during the radiographic procedure EXCEPT one. Which one is the EXCEPTION?

    A. Request that the patient concentrate on the image receptor being placed intraorally.
    B. Direct the patient to raise one leg or wiggle a finger during the radiographic procedure.
    C. Ask the patient to hold his or her breath or hum a song while the image receptor is being placed intraorally.
    D. Ensure that the patient is pressing the back of his or her head against the chair's headrest during the radiographic procedure.

4. When exposing a maxillary periapical radiograph on a patient with a large palatine torus, where should the image receptor be placed?

    A. In front of the torus
    B. Behind the torus
    C. On top of the torus
    D. Touching the torus

5. When exposing a mandibular periapical radiograph on a patient with large mandibular tori, where should the image receptor be placed?

    A. In front of the tori
    B. Behind the tori
    C. On top of the tori
    D. On top of the tongue

6. Each of the following is considered an appropriate action to help facilitate placement of an image receptor when the patient exhibits a large, tight mandibular frenulum EXCEPT one. Which one is the EXCEPTION?

    A. Massage the sublingual area.
    B. Shield the alveolar mucosa with a finger.
    C. Rest the image receptor on the tongue.
    D. Request that the patient close halfway.

7. Which of the following adjustments may be indicated for an edentulous area?
   A. Decrease the exposure time.
   B. Decrease the vertical angulation of the x-ray beam.
   C. Increase the distance between the image receptor and alveolar ridge.
   D. Increase the kilovoltage setting.

8. Each of the following is a reason to alter radiographic techniques for the child patient EXCEPT one. Which one is the EXCEPTION?
   A. Small oral cavity
   B. Lack of tongue control
   C. Increased oral sensitivity
   D. Poor self-care

9. Which of the following adjustments to basic radiographic techniques may be required to appropriately image areas with malaligned teeth?
   A. Increase the number of radiographs exposed.
   B. Increase the milliamperage setting.
   C. Decrease the vertical angulation of the x-ray beam.
   D. Decrease the size of the image receptor.

10. Reflect on your experience today. Having experienced the radiographic procedure as a patient, what insights have you gathered about the procedure? Did you experience anything today that would prompt you to adjust your management of patients in the future?

_____

_____

_____

_____

_____

_____

_____

_____

_____

Occlusal Radiographic Techniques

INTRODUCTION

Developing the skills required for obtaining diagnostic quality occlusal radiographs will round out the dental radiographer's working knowledge of intraoral radiographic techniques. Occlusal radiographs can play a valuable role in diagnosis and planning treatment for both adults and children. Occlusal radiographs usually use a size #4 image receptor for adults and a size #2 image receptor for children. The larger image receptor size, when combined with the occlusal technique, records a larger area of information than may be recorded on smaller-sized image receptors usually used for periapical radiographs. The value of occlusal radiographs is the ability to detect supernumerary, unerupted, or impacted teeth; record areas of large pathology such as a cyst or tumor; locate retained roots or foreign bodies; evaluate tooth or jaw fractures; and reveal the presence of soft tissue diseases or conditions such as salivary stones. Occlusal radiographs may aid in examining patients who cannot tolerate placement of a periapical radiograph. The purpose of this exercise is to introduce the techniques used for obtaining occlusal radiographs.

OBJECTIVES

Following completion of this lab activity, you will be able to:

1. Demonstrate proficiency in placing, exposing, and processing topographical occlusal radiographs.

2. Demonstrate proficiency in placing, exposing, and processing cross-sectional occlusal radiographs.

3. Identify the buccal/lingual positions of objects radiographically through interpretation of an occlusal radiographic image.

MATERIALS

Teaching manikin or skull

Lead/lead equivalent apron with thyroid collar

Size #4 radiographic films (or photostimuable phosphor [PSP] plates if available)

Size #2 radiographic films (or photostimuable phosphor [PSP] plates if available)

Periapical image receptor holding device

Metal object or sample extracted tooth

Red sticky wax or similar adhesive material

Viewbox

PREPARATION

1. Study the chapter outline to prepare for this laboratory exercise. An understanding of the material presented in the outline is required to complete this activity.

2. Utilize Table 10–1 to assist you with completing the exercise. Instructor demonstration may enhance knowledge of the laboratory activity.

3. Prepare radiology operatory. Set up teaching manikin or skull. Ensure that correct "patient" positioning is achieved for the type of projection you are exposing. To image the maxilla, ensure that the maxillary occlusal plane is parallel to the floor; to image the mandible, ensure that the mandibular occlusal plane is parallel to the floor and the midsagittal plane must be perpendicular to the floor for both maxillary and mandibular exposures. Tip the patient's head back so that the occlusal plane is perpendicular to the floor for the mandibular cross-sectional occlusal radiographs

4. Place lead/lead equivalent apron and thyroid collar over the "patient."

LABORATORY EXERCISE ACTIVITIES

Part 1: Occlusal Radiographs

1. Obtain five size #4 radiographic film packets. (If available, size #4 photostimuable phosphor [PSP] plates may be used for this activity.)

2. Check posted exposure settings for the dental x-ray machine and set for occlusal radiographs. (If no settings for occlusal radiographs are posted, use the settings for periapical radiographs in that region.)

3. Using Table 10–1, place and expose the following occlusal radiographs:
   a. Maxillary anterior topographical occlusal radiograph
   b. Maxillary posterior topographical occlusal radiograph (choose either the right or the left side)
   c. Mandibular anterior topographical occlusal radiograph
   d. Mandibular posterior topographical occlusal radiograph (choose either the right or the left side)

TABLE 10–1 Summary of Steps for Acquiring Occlusal Radiographs

Occlusal Radiograph	Packet Placement	Vertical Angulation*	Horizontal Angulation	Centering*
Maxillary Topographical (anterior)	Long dimension across the mouth (buccal-to-buccal). White unprinted film side toward the maxillary teeth.	Perpendicular to the imaginary bisector between the long axes of the teeth and the image receptor in the vertical dimension; +65 degrees (Figure 10–1 ■).	Perpendicular to the image receptor through the maxillary central incisor embrasure.	Through a point near the bridge of the nose toward the center of the image receptor.
Maxillary Topographical (posterior)	Long dimension along the midline (front-to-back). White unprinted film side toward the maxillary teeth.	Perpendicular to the imaginary bisector between the long axes of the teeth and the image receptor in the vertical dimension; +45 degrees (Figure 10–2 ■).	Perpendicular to the image receptor through the maxillary posterior embrasures.	Through a point on the ala-tragus line below the outer canthus of the eye toward the center of the image receptor.
Mandibular Topographical (anterior)	Long dimension across the mouth (buccal-to-buccal). White unprinted film side toward the mandibular teeth.	Perpendicular to the imaginary bisector between the long axes of the teeth and the image receptor in the vertical dimension; –55 degrees (Figure 10–3 ■).	Perpendicular to the image receptor through the mandibular central incisor embrasure.	Through a point on the middle of the chin toward the center of the image receptor.
Mandibular Topographical (posterior)	Long dimension along the midline (front-to-back). White unprinted film side toward the mandibular teeth.	Perpendicular to the imaginary bisector between the long axes of the teeth and the image receptor in the vertical dimension; –45 degrees (Figure 10–4 ■).	Perpendicular to the image receptor through the mandibular posterior embrasures.	Through a point on the inferior border of the mandible directly below the second mandibular premolar toward the center of the image receptor.
Mandibular Cross-sectional	Long dimension across the mouth (buccal-to-buccal). White unprinted film side toward the mandibular teeth.	Perpendicular to the image receptor; 0 degrees (Figure 10–5 ■).	Align the open end of the PID parallel to the plane of the image receptor.	Through a point 2 in. (5 cm) back from the tip of the chin toward the center of the image receptor.

*The patient must be seated in the correct position with the occlusal plane of the arch being imaged parallel to the floor (for topographic occlusal radiographs) or the chin up and the head tilted back as far as possible to align the occlusal plane perpendicular to the floor (for cross-sectional occlusal radiographs) and the midsagittal plane perpendicular to the floor to use the vertical angulation and points of entry recommended in this chart.

Reference: Thomson, E. M., & Johnson, O.N. (2012). *Essentials of dental radiography for dental assistants and hygienists* (9th ed.). Upper Saddle River, NJ: Pearson.

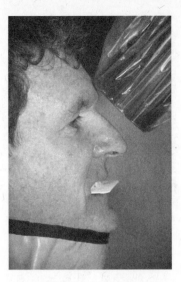

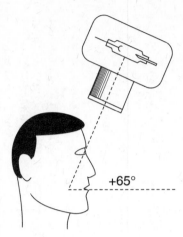

Figure 10–1 Vertical angulation required for the maxillary anterior topographical occlusal radiograph.

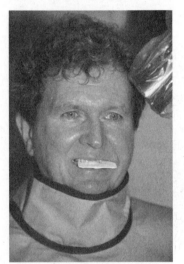

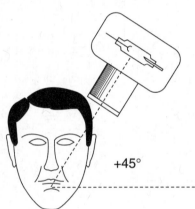

Figure 10–2 Vertical angulation required for the maxillary posterior topographical occlusal radiograph.

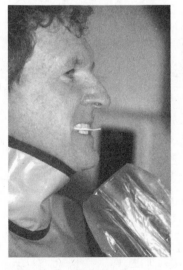

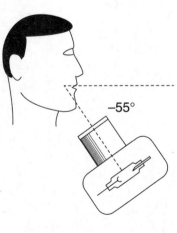

Figure 10–3 Vertical angulation required for the mandibular anterior topographical occlusal radiograph.

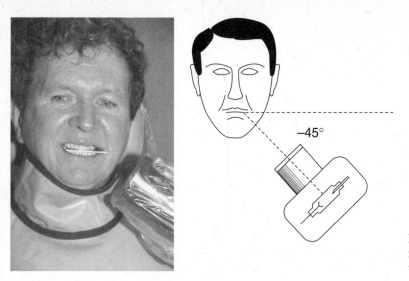

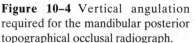

−45°

Figure 10–4 Vertical angulation required for the mandibular posterior topographical occlusal radiograph.

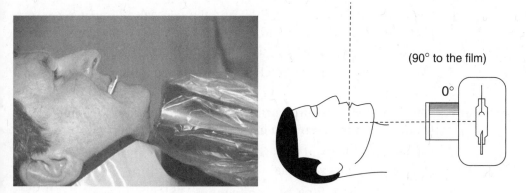

(90° to the film)

0°

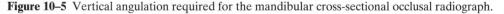

Figure 10–5 Vertical angulation required for the mandibular cross-sectional occlusal radiograph.

      e.   Mandibular cross-sectional occlusal radiograph (reposition the "patient's" head by tipping the chin up)

  4. Process the five films or scan the PSP plates.

Part 2: Right-angle Method of Localization Using Occlusal Radiographs

1. Using red sticky wax or other adhesive, attach an extracted molar or metal object to the teaching manikin or skull on the buccal side of the right mandibular first molar region (Figure 10–6 ■) and the lingual side of the left mandibular first molar region. Center the objects in the middle of the furcation area of the first molars. These objects will simulate an impaction or foreign object.

2. Obtain two size #2 and one size #4 radiographic film packets. (If available, size #2 and size #4 PSP plates may be used for this activity.)

3. Check the posted exposure settings for the dental x-ray machine and set for mandibular posterior periapical radiographs.

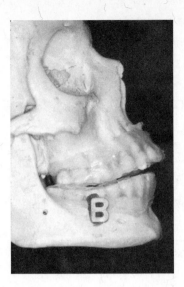

Figure 10–6 A metal object is attached to the teaching manikin with sticky wax to simulate the presence of a foreign body.

4. Using an image receptor holder and the two size #2 image receptors, place and expose the mandibular right and the mandibular left molar periapical radiographs utilizing the paralleling technique. Set aside.

5. Reposition the patient's head for exposing a mandibular cross-sectional occlusal radiograph.

6. Check posted exposure settings for the dental x-ray machine, and set for the mandibular cross-sectional occlusal radiograph.

7. Using Table 10–1 and the size #4 image receptor, place and expose the mandibular cross-sectional occlusal radiograph.

8. Process the three films or scan the three PSP plates.

COMPETENCY AND EVALUATION

1. Mount the processed radiographs on the simulated film mounts that follow. Secure with a piece of tape placed along the top edge of the radiograph only, so that it may be raised slightly, to allow light underneath for ease of viewing. Using removable transparent tape will allow the film mount page to be used more than once. (If using digital technology, observe the images on the computer monitor or print out a copy of the images at the direction of your instructor.)
   NOTE: Use the labial mounting method. (See Laboratory Exercise 6, Film Mounting and Radiographic Landmarks, for details.) The raised portion of the embossed dot is toward you (convex) when placing the radiograph onto the page.

2. Place the page with the mounted radiographs taped to it on a viewbox and evaluate for acceptability. Based on the four steps: packet placement, vertical and horizontal angulation, and centering the PID, what is the quality of the images? Are the correct teeth imaged? Is there elongation or foreshortening error? Is the area of interest overlapped? Is there conecut error? Does the conecut affect an important part of the image? Why would conecut error be acceptable in the anterior

region of the image? What steps would you take to improve your skills in taking occlusal radiographs? Obtain instructor feedback. Identify which step (packet placement, vertical angulation, horizontal angulation, centering) needs improvement. Repeat Part 1 at the direction of your instructor. The film mount page may be copied to accommodate multiple practice attempts to achieve competency.

3. Describe the difference in appearance between the image obtained utilizing the topographical technique and the cross-sectional technique. What conditions might the patient present with that would prompt the dentist to prescribe a topographical occlusal radiograph? A cross-sectional occlusal radiograph? Describe the role the cross-sectional occlusal radiograph plays in locating buccal-lingual objects radiographically. Why would it be difficult to use occlusal radiographs to locate objects on the maxilla? If you did not know where these objects were attached, how would you be able to tell the buccal or lingual location by examining these radiographs?

4. Complete the study questions.

Part 1: Occlusal Radiographs

Maxillary Anterior Topographical

Maxillary Posterior Topographical

Mandibular Anterior Topographical

Mandibular Posterior Topographical

Mandibular Cross-sectional

Part 2: Right-angle Localization Method

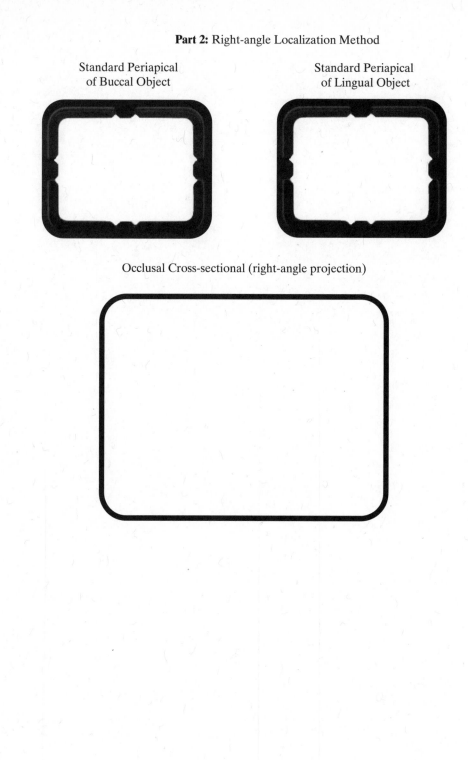

Standard Periapical
of Buccal Object

Standard Periapical
of Lingual Object

Occlusal Cross-sectional (right-angle projection)

I. Occlusal radiographs
   A. Purpose
      1. Records a larger area than periapical radiographs (if using a size #4 image receptor)
      2. Can be used as an acceptable substitute when the patient cannot tolerate intraoral placement of periapical radiographs (Figure 10–7 ■)
         a. Children
         b. Patients with a low, sensitive palatal vault
         c. Patients with an exaggerated gag reflex
         d. Patients who are unable to open due to fractures or temporomandibular disorder (TMD)
      3. Can be used as an aid in locating the buccal or lingual position of foreign objects, impactions, or supernumerary teeth, cysts, or other conditions
   B. Types
      1. Topographical occlusal radiograph
         a. Image produced resembles a large periapical radiograph (Figure 10–8 ■)
         b. Useful for examinations in the anterior or posterior of both the maxilla and mandible
      2. Cross-sectional occlusal radiograph
         a. Image produced superimposes the apical and occlusal regions, resulting in tooth structures that resemble a circular or elliptical appearance (Figure 10–8)
         b. Due to the increased thickness of the facial structures of the maxilla and superior skull, more useful for examinations in the anterior or posterior of mandible than the maxilla
         c. Often used to examine sublingual (under the tongue) soft tissues for calcifications or foreign bodies
         d. Valuable in determining the buccal or lingual location of impacted or supernumerary teeth, cysts, and foreign bodies.
   C. Examinations—may be taken in any region of the oral cavity. Most common placements are:
      1. Maxillary topographical (anterior)
      2. Maxillary topographical (posterior)

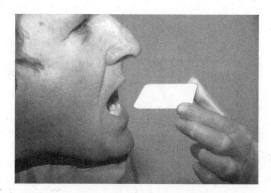

Figure 10–7 The occlusal image receptor placement is easily tolerated by the patient with a low, sensitive palatal vault.

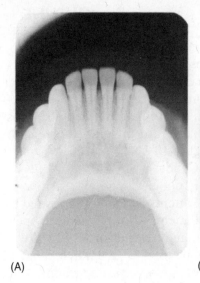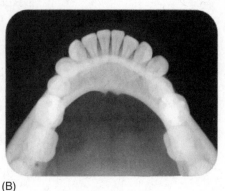

(A)   (B)

Figure 10–8 (A) Topographical occlusal radiograph of the anterior mandible. (B) Cross-sectional occlusal radiograph of the anterior mandible.

  3. Mandibular topographical (anterior)
  4. Mandibular topographical (posterior)
  5. Mandibular cross-sectional
 D. Principal concepts
  1. A size #4 image receptor is used to expose occlusal radiographs for adult patients.
  2. A size #2 image receptor is used to expose occlusal radiographs for children or for adults in situations that call for a smaller, limited recording region.
  3. An image receptor holder is not required. The patient holds the image receptor in position by lightly occluding directly on the image receptor.
  4. The technique is based on the bisecting technique, where the central ray of the x-ray beam is directed perpendicular to the imaginary bisector between the long axes of the teeth and the plane of the image receptor.
  5. The white, unprinted side of the film packet is placed toward the arch being imaged. When using a phosphor plate, determine the front side by reading the instructions printed on the plate by the manufacturer. Currently, digital sensors are not available in size #4 for occlusal radiographs on adult patients.
  6. The embossed dot on film-based image receptors is placed away from the area of interest (toward the anterior) (Figure 10–9 ■).
  7. The image receptor should extend at least 1/4 inch beyond the anterior teeth of the arch image imaged (Figure 10–9).
  8. Dental x-ray machine settings should be based on the manufacturer's recommendations; usually the same settings as those indicated for periapical radiographs in the same region.
 E. Maxillary and mandibular anterior and posterior topographical occlusal radiographs—see Table 10–1
  1. Patient is seated upright with occlusal plane parallel to the floor and the midsagittal plane perpendicular to the floor

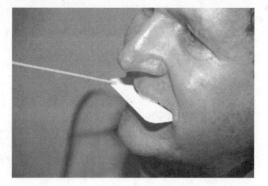

Figure 10–9 The embossed dot is placed anteriorly and the image receptor is extending at least one-fourth inch beyond the maxillary anterior teeth, indicating correct maxillary topographical occlusal film packet placement.

2. Image receptor is positioned with the longer dimension across the patient's right and left sides for anterior views or with the longer dimension front-to-back for posterior views.

F. Mandibular anterior and posterior cross-sectional occlusal radiographs—see Table 10–1
  1. Patient is seated upright with the chin up and the head tilted back as far as possible to align the occlusal plane perpendicular to the floor.
  2. The image receptor is positioned with the longer dimension across the patient's right and left sides for anterior views or with the longer dimension front-to-back for posterior views.

G. Criteria for diagnostic quality
  1. Area of interest is accurately recorded.
  2. There is no overlapping of the proximal surfaces.
  3. Image is free of distortion (elongation or foreshortening).
  4. Conecutting is absent or minimal. (If conecutting occurs, it should be confined to the anterior region where the image is least likely to be affected.)
  5. The embossed dot should be away from the image area, positioned toward the anterior region.

II. Interpreting occlusal radiographs for buccal/lingual positions of objects
  A. If an object has been identified on a periapical radiograph, an additional exposure using the cross-sectional occlusal technique (called a right-angle projection when used in localization methods) can reveal the object's buccal or lingual position (Figure 10–10 ■).

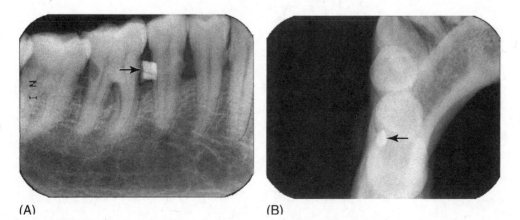

(A) (B)

Figure 10–10 (A) Radiopaque foreign object identified on a periapical radiograph. (B) Occlusal cross-sectional radiograph of this same region reveals that the object is located in a buccal position.

B. Occlusal radiographs are more effective on the mandible than the maxilla. The presence of multiple thick bones of the maxillary region limit the ability of a cross-sectional occlusal radiograph to image details of the teeth and surrounding bone.

REFERENCES

O'Carroll, M. K. (1993). *Advanced radiographic techniques part I: Occlusal and lateral oblique projections.* Study guide to videotape series. Chapel Hill, NC: Health Sciences Consortium.

Thomson, E. M., & Johnson, O. N. (2012). *Essentials of dental radiography for dental assistants and hygienists* (9th ed.). Upper Saddle River, NJ: Pearson,

1. Occlusal radiographs are useful for each of the following EXCEPT one. Which one is the EXCEPTION?
    A. Examining the severity of periodontal disease
    B. Locating supernumerary teeth
    C. Determining extent of fractures
    D. Evaluating salivary gland stones
    E. Imaging large pathological lesions

2. The occlusal radiograph may be substituted when a child patient cannot tolerate placement of a periapical image receptor.

    A size #2 image receptor may be used when taking occlusal radiographs on a child.
    A. The first statement is true. The second statement is false.
    B. The first statement is false. The second statement is true.
    C. Both statements are true.
    D. Both statements are false.

3. Which of the following projections would best image an unexplained sublingual swelling?
    A. Topographical occlusal radiograph
    B. Cross-sectional occlusal radiograph

4. Which of the following projections would best evaluate delayed eruption of the maxillary lateral incisors in a child patient?
    A. Topographical occlusal radiograph
    B. Cross-sectional occlusal radiograph

5. Which of the following image receptor sizes would most likely be used to expose an occlusal radiograph on an adult patient?
    A. #0
    B. #1
    C. #2
    D. #3
    E. #4

6. When placing a film-based image receptor for an occlusal radiograph, the embossed dot should be positioned toward the _____ of the oral cavity.
    A. mesial
    B. distal
    C. posterior
    D. anterior

7. Which of the following occlusal radiographs requires that the patient's head be positioned tipped back with the chin up and the occlusal plane vertical to the floor?
    A. Maxillary topographical (anterior)
    B. Maxillary topographical (posterior)
    C. Mandibular topographical (anterior)
    D. Mandibular topographical (posterior)
    E. Mandibular cross-sectional

8. To determine the vertical angulation for a mandibular cross-sectional occlusal radiograph, the central ray of the x-ray beam is directed
    A. Perpendicular to the imaginary bisector.
    B. Parallel to the imaginary bisector.
    C. Perpendicular to the image receptor.
    D. Parallel to the image receptor.

9. Referring to the previous question and assuming the patient's head position is correct, at which of the following angles would the PID most likely be set?
    A. +65 degrees
    B. +45 degrees
    C. −55 degrees
    D. 0 degrees

10. Which of the following would result in a retake of a maxillary topographical radiograph?
    A. Long dimension of image receptor positioned across the arch buccal-to-buccal
    B. Conecutting in the posterior
    C. Embossed dot positioned toward the anterior
    D. Image receptor positioned such that 1/4 inch protrudes beyond the incisal edges

laboratory exercise 11

Supplemental Radiographic Techniques and Tips

INTRODUCTION

A dental radiographer must possess the knowledge and skills to perform basic oral radiographic techniques. What sets the exceptional dental radiographer apart is the ability to adapt techniques to perform advanced radiographic services for the patient. Theory provides the knowledge base that guides radiographic practice, but acceptable deviations from the basic techniques, when implemented correctly, can obtain radiographs in situations that might have made radiographs unobtainable. In addition to acquiring quality radiographs under less than ideal conditions, the dental radiographer trained in advanced techniques can interpret the maximum amount of information from radiographs.

The purpose of this exercise is to introduce tips for achieving diagnostic quality radiographs in special situations. Practicing these skills and evaluating the resulting images will complete the competent dental radiographer's skill set.

OBJECTIVES

Following completion of this lab activity, you will be able to:

1. Demonstrate proficiency in placing, exposing, and processing disto-oblique periapical radiographs.

2. Demonstrate proficiency in utilizing localization to enhance radiographic interpretation.

3. Apply acceptable deviations from standard techniques when presented with unique situations.

MATERIALS

Teaching manikin or skull

Lead/lead equivalent apron with thyroid collar

Size #2 radiographic films or photostimuable phosphor (PSP) plates

Size #2 digital sensor

Periapical image receptor holding device

Metal object or sample extracted tooth

Lead letters "M," "D," "O," and "A" or 4 different metal objects for labeling

Red sticky wax or similar adhesive material

Viewbox

PREPARATION

1. Study the chapter outline to prepare for this laboratory exercise. An understanding of the material presented in the outline is required to complete this activity.

2. Use Table 11–1 to assist you with completing the exercise. Instructor demonstration may enhance knowledge of the laboratory exercise.

3. Prepare radiology operatory. Set up teaching manikin or skull. Ensure that correct "patient" positioning is achieved for the type of projection you are exposing. To image the maxilla, ensure that the maxillary occlusal plane is parallel to the floor; to image the mandible, ensure that the mandibular occlusal plane is parallel to the floor and the midsagittal plane must be perpendicular to the floor for both maxillary and mandibular exposures.

4. Place lead/lead equivalent apron and thyroid collar over the "patient."

LABORATORY EXERCISE ACTIVITIES

Part 1: Disto-oblique Periapical Radiographs

1. Use the patient's right side for this activity. Using red sticky wax or other adhesive, attach an extracted tooth or metal object to the teaching manikin or skull in the area of the maxillary tuberosity (Figure 11–1 ■) and in the region of the mandibular retromolar pad (Figure 11–2 ■). This object will simulate a posteriorly located impaction or foreign object.

2. Obtain four size #2 radiographic film packets or photostimuable phosphor (PSP) plates. A size #2 digital sensor may be used if available.

3. Check the posted exposure settings for the dental x-ray machine and set for a maxillary molar periapical radiograph.

TABLE 11-1 Disto-oblique Periapical Radiographs

Maxillary Disto-oblique Periapical Radiograph	Mandibular Disto-oblique Periapical Radiograph
Position the image receptor as far posterior as possible.	Position the image receptor as far posterior as possible.
Align the PID into the correct vertical and horizontal angles for a standard periapical radiograph. Center the image receptor in the middle of the x-ray beam.	Align the PID into the correct vertical and horizontal angles for a standard periapical radiograph. Center the image receptor in the middle of the x-ray beam.
Alter the horizontal angulation by shifting the PID so that the x-ray beam will intersect the image receptor obliquely 10 degrees from the distal.	Alter the horizontal angulation by shifting the PID so that the x-ray beam will intersect the image receptor obliquely 10 degrees from the distal.
Increase the vertical angulation 5 degrees over standard.	Do not change the vertical angulation from standard.
Increase the exposure time by one setting over standard.	Do not change the exposure time from standard.

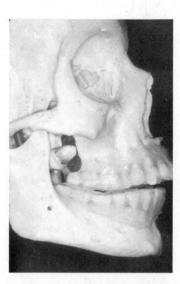

Figure 11–1 A posteriorly located "impacted" maxillary molar is attached to the teaching manikin with sticky wax.

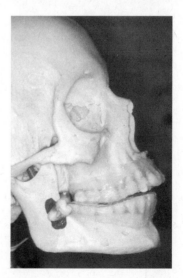

Figure 11–2 A posteriorly located "impacted" mandibular molar is attached to the teaching manikin with sticky wax.

4. Using an image receptor holder and the paralleling technique, place the first image receptor into the standard position for exposing the maxillary right molar periapical. (Note that this standard position will *not* image the posteriorly located impacted molar or metal object. This would be especially true if this patient had a hypersensitive gag reflex, which would prevent posterior placement of the image receptor.)

5. Expose the standard maxillary molar periapical and set aside. If using direct digital technology, save this first image before proceeding and do not move the sensor.

6. Next, using the paralleling technique, place the second image receptor into the exact same standard position for exposing the maxillary right molar periapical. If using direct digital technology, do not move the sensor. (Again, this standard position will not image the posteriorly located "impacted" molar or metal object.) Use Table 11–1 to adjust the horizontal and vertical angulations and the timer setting to expose a disto-oblique periapical radiograph of this maxillary region and set aside. If using direct digital technology, save this second image.

7. Next, check the posted exposure settings for the dental x-ray machine and set for a mandibular molar periapical radiograph.

8. Repeat steps 4, 5, and 6 using Table 11–1 to expose a disto-oblique periapical radiograph of the mandibular region.

9. Process the four films or scan the PSP plates. If using direct digital technology, observe the four images on the computer monitor.

Part 2: Demonstration of the Tube-shift Method of Localization

1. Use the patient's left side for this activity. Using red sticky wax or other adhesive, attach an extracted tooth or metal object to the teaching manikin or skull on the lingual surface of the maxillary left first molar region and to the buccal surface of the mandibular left first molar region (see Figure 10–6).

2. Obtain ten size #2 radiographic image receptors. A size #2 digital sensor may be used if available.

3. Check the posted exposure settings for the dental x-ray machine and set for maxillary posterior periapical radiographs.

4. Obtain a periapical image receptor holder. Use a device such as a Stabe® without an extension arm and aiming device since these may get in the way when altering the angulation of the PID.

5. Use one of the size #2 image receptors to place and expose a standard maxillary left molar periapical radiograph utilizing the paralleling technique. Set aside. If using direct digital technology, save the image before proceeding.

6. Next, using four of the remaining size #2 image receptors, place each in the same position to expose the maxillary left molar. The image receptor position should be the same as the standard placement, only now you will be shifting the PID from standard alignment. Using sticky

wax, label each of the four image receptors with a lead letter so that you will be able to identify which image was taken with which shift in the PID alignment. Place the lead letter near the edge of the image receptor to position it out of the way (Figure 11–3 ■).

7. Shift the PID horizontally and vertically, into the following four positions for each of the four exposures on the maxillary left side. Shift the PID:

    a. Horizontally, so that the x-ray beam will strike the image receptor obliquely 10 degrees from the mesial. (Label image receptor with the lead letter "M" to indicate a mesial shift.) (Figure 11–4 ■)

    b. Horizontally, so that the x-ray beam will strike the image receptor obliquely 10 degrees from the distal. (Label image receptor with the lead letter "D" to indicate a distal shift.) (Figure 11–5 ■)

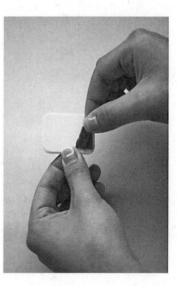

Figure 11–3 Labeling the film packet by attaching a lead letter with sticky wax.

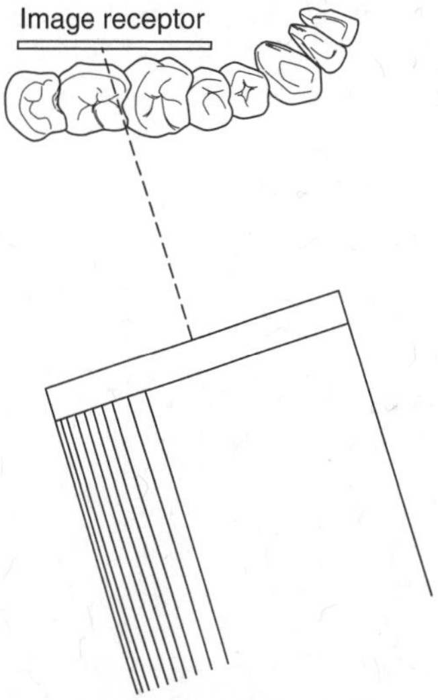

Image receptor

Figure 11–4 Demonstration of the tube-shift method of localization. Alter the horizontal angulation approximately 10 degrees from the mesial.

c. Vertically, so that the x-ray beam will strike the image receptor obliquely 10 degrees from the occlusal plane. (Label image receptor with the lead letter "O" to indicate an occlusal shift.) (Figure 11–6 ■)

d. Vertically, so that the x-ray beam will strike the image receptor obliquely 10 degrees from the apical region. (Label image receptor with the lead letter "A" to indicate an apical shift.) (Figure 11–7 ■)

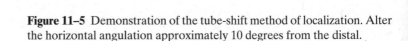

Figure 11–5 Demonstration of the tube-shift method of localization. Alter the horizontal angulation approximately 10 degrees from the distal.

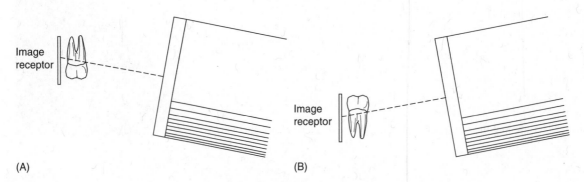

(A) (B)

Figure 11–6 Demonstration of the tube-shift method of localization. Alter the vertical angulation approximately 10 degrees from the occlusal (A) maxilla and (B) mandible.

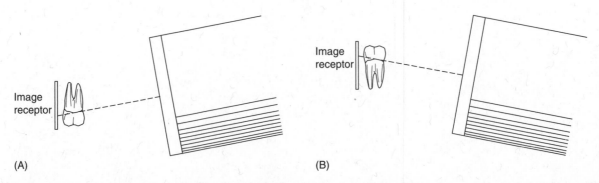

(A) (B)

Figure 11–7 Demonstration of the tube-shift method of localization. Alter the vertical angulation approximately 10 degrees from the apical (A) maxilla and (B) mandible.

8. Set the five exposures aside. If using direct digital technology, save the five images before proceeding.

9. Obtain an additional five image receptors and repeat steps 5, 6, and 7 with each of the five exposures on the mandibular left side.

10. Process all ten films or scan the PSP plates. If using direct digital technology, observe the ten images on the computer monitor.

Part 3: Radiographic Technique Tips for Unique Situations

1. Maxillary molar overlap
    a. Obtain two size #2 radiographic film packets or PSP plates. A size #2 digital sensor may be used if available.
    b. Check the posted exposure settings for the dental x-ray machine and set for a maxillary molar periapical radiograph.
    c. Using an image receptor holder and the paralleling technique, place the first image receptor into the standard position for exposing the maxillary right molar periapical radiograph. Expose and set aside. If using direct digital technology, save the image before proceeding.
    d. Next, using the paralleling technique, place the second image receptor into position for exposing the maxillary right molar periapical radiograph using the radiographic technique tip for overcoming maxillary molar overlap (Figure 11–8 ■).
    e. Process the two films or scan the two PSP plates. If using digital technology, observe the two images on the computer monitor.

2. Canine-first premolar overlap
    a. Obtain two size #1 radiographic film packets or PSP plates. A size #1 digital sensor may be used if available.
    b. Check the posted exposure settings for the dental x-ray machine and set for a maxillary canine periapical radiograph.
    c. Using an image receptor holder and the paralleling technique, place the first image receptor into the standard position for exposing the maxillary right canine radiograph. Expose and set aside. If using direct digital technology, save the image before proceeding.
    d. Next, using the paralleling technique, place the second image receptor into position for exposing the maxillary right canine periapical radiograph using the radiographic technique tip for overcoming canine-first premolar overlap (Figure 11–9 ■).
    e. Process the two films or scan the two PSP plates. If using direct digital technology, observe the two images on the computer monitor.

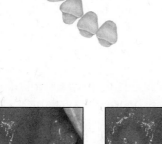

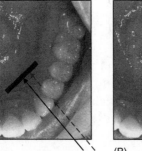

Figure 11–8 Positioning the anterior edge of the image receptor a greater distance from the lingual surfaces of the teeth aligns the image receptor more accurately perpendicular to the interproximal space between the first and second maxillary molars.

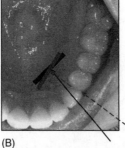

(A)   (B)

Figure 11–9 (A) Standard image receptor and horizontal angulation position. (B) Shifting the image receptor position and the horizontal angulation to eliminate overlap of the distal portion of the canine with the mesial portion of the lingual cusp of the first premolar.

3. Not recording the distal edge of the maxillary and mandibular canines on a premolar bitewing radiograph.

     a. Obtain two size #2 radiographic film packets or PSP plates. A size #2 digital sensor may be used if available.

     b. Check the posted exposure settings for the dental x-ray machine and set for a premolar bitewing radiograph.

    c.   Using an image receptor holder and the bitewing technique, place the first image receptor into the standard position for exposing the right premolar bitewing radiograph. Expose and set aside. If using direct digital technology, save the image before proceeding.

    d.   Next, using the bitewing technique, place the second image receptor into position for exposing the right premolar bitewing radiograph using the radiographic technique tip for overcoming not recording the distal edge of the maxillary and mandibular canines on a premolar bitewing radiograph (Figure 11–10 ■).

    e.   Process the two films or scan the two PSP plates. If using direct digital technology, observe the two images on the computer monitor.

4. Not recording the incisal edges of the teeth of interest

    a.   Obtain two size #2 radiographic film packets or PSP plates. A size #2 digital sensor may be used if available.

    b.   Check the posted exposure settings for the dental x-ray machine and set for a maxillary central incisor periapical radiograph.

    c.   Using an image receptor holder and the paralleling technique, place the first image receptor into the standard position for exposing the maxillary central incisor radiograph. Expose and set aside. If using direct digital technology, save the image before proceeding and do not move the sensor.

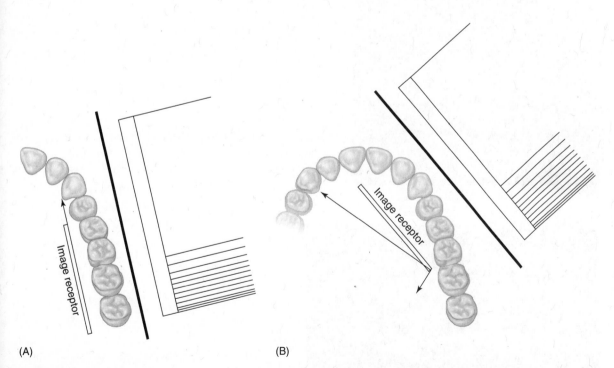

(A)   (B)

Figure 11–10 (A) Sliding this image receptor anteriorally may not record the distal portion of the canines on both the maxilla and the mandible. (B) Image receptor positioned away from the lingual surfaces of the teeth and moved anterior to contact the lingual surface of the canine on the opposite side. The posterior edge of the image receptor is also moved away from the lingual surfaces of the teeth to avoid overlap error in this altered position.

d. Next, using the paralleling technique, place the second image receptor into position for exposing the maxillary central incisor periapical radiograph using the radiographic technique tip for overcoming not recording the incisal edges of the teeth of interest (Figure 11–11 ■). If using direct digital technology the sensor will already be in position.

5. Not recording the apices of the teeth of interest

   a. Obtain two size #2 radiographic film packets or PSP plates. A size #2 digital sensor may be used if available.

   b. Check the posted exposure settings for the dental x-ray machine and set for a maxillary right molar periapical radiograph.

   c. Using an image receptor holder and the paralleling technique, place the first image receptor into the standard position for exposing the maxillary right molar periapical radiograph. Expose and set aside. If using direct digital technology, save the image before proceeding and do not move the sensor.

   d. Next, using the paralleling technique, place the second image receptor into position for exposing the maxillary right molar periapical radiograph using the radiographic technique tip for overcoming not recording the apices of the teeth of interest (Figure 11–12 ■). If using direct digital technology the sensor will already be in position.

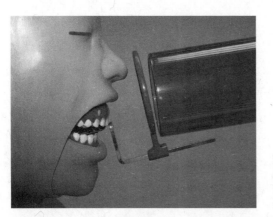

Figure 11–11 PID in correct position to image the incisal edges of the anterior teeth. Note that the reduction in vertical angulation is less than 15 degrees from that indicated by the external aiming ring on this image receptor holder.

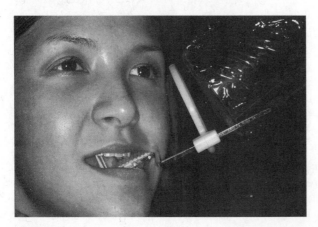

Figure 11–12 Increasing the vertical angulation will record more of the periapical region. Note that the PID is not aimed directly at the external aiming ring of the image receptor holder.

6. Unequal distribution of the arches recorded on bitewing radiographs

    a. Obtain two size #2 radiographic film packets or PSP plates. A size #2 digital sensor may be used if available.

    b. Check the posted exposure settings for the dental x-ray machine and set for a molar bitewing radiograph.

    c. Using an image receptor holder and the bitewing technique, place the first image receptor into the standard position for exposing the right molar bitewing radiograph. Expose and set aside. If using direct digital technology, save the image before proceeding.

    d. Next, using the bitewing technique, place the second image receptor into position for exposing the right molar bitewing radiograph using the radiographic technique tip for overcoming inadequate distribution of the arches recorded on bitewing radiographs (Figure 11–13 ■).

COMPETENCY AND EVALUATION

1. Mount the processed radiographs on the simulated film mounts that follow. Secure with a piece of tape placed along the top edge of the radiograph only, so that the radiographs may be raised slightly, to allow light underneath for ease of viewing.

   Note: Use the labial mounting method. (See Laboratory Exercise 6, Film Mounting and Radiographic Landmarks, for details.) The raised portion of the embossed dot is toward you (convex) when placing the film onto the page. (If using digital technology, observe the images on the computer monitor or print out a copy of the images at the direction of your instructor.)

2. Place the simulated mount pages on a viewbox and evaluate. Obtain instructor feedback.

3. Examine the resultant radiographic images in each of the three parts of this exercise. Based on your results, summarize the following in your own words:

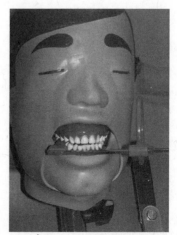

Figure 11–13 Alternate assembly allows the patient to occlude on the opposite side preventing long maxillary facial cusps from forcing the image receptor holder down into an inadequate vertical angulation.

a. Part 1 Disto-oblique periapical radiographs
Compare the standard and disto-oblique periapical radiographs side-by-side. Is the disto-oblique image a reasonable representation of the anatomical structures? Is image distortion minimal? Describe the difference between the two images. Did the disto-oblique periapical radiograph record structures that were located further posterior than the standard image receptor placement did? What is the advantage to this? What conditions might the patient present with that would prompt the dentist to prescribe a disto-oblique periapical radiograph?

b. Part 2 Demonstration of the tube-shift method of localization
If these objects were hidden under the patient's soft tissues, and you did not know where these objects were attached, how would you be able to tell the buccal or lingual location by examining these radiographs? When examining the radiographs of the maxillary molar region, what can you summarize about the direction the attached object appeared to "move" in? When examining the radiographs of the mandibular molar region, what can you summarize about the direction the attached object appeared to "move" in? Explain how you would utilize your knowledge of the tube-shift method of locating an object imaged in two places on a full mouth or bitewing series.

c. Part 3 Radiographic technique tips for unique situations
Compare the standard radiograph exposed first with the second radiograph exposed using the radiographic technique tips for unique situations. Did the radiographic technique tip help with improving the diagnostic quality of the images? Did additional errors occur with when using the tip? If so, what do you think is the reason? How do you think you will utilize these tips with patients?

4. Complete the study questions.

Part 1: Disto-oblique Periapical Radiographs

Maxillary Standard Periapical   Maxillary Disto-oblique Periapical

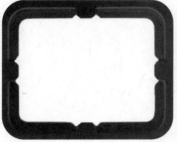 

Mandibular Standard Periapical   Mandibular Disto-oblique Periapical

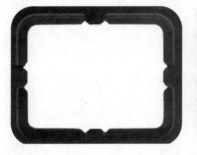 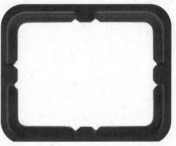

Part 2: Tube Shift Method of Localization—Lingual Location

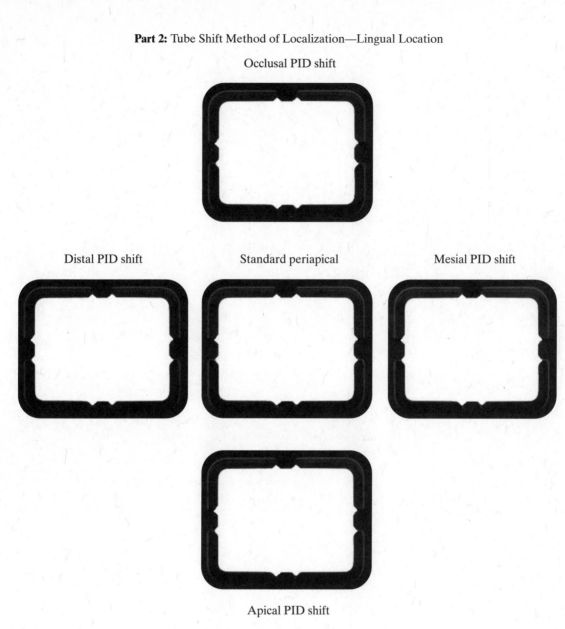

Occlusal PID shift

Distal PID shift   Standard periapical   Mesial PID shift

Apical PID shift

Supplemental Radiographic Techniques and Tips   **267**

Part 2: Tube Shift Method of Localization—Buccal Location

Occlusal PID shift

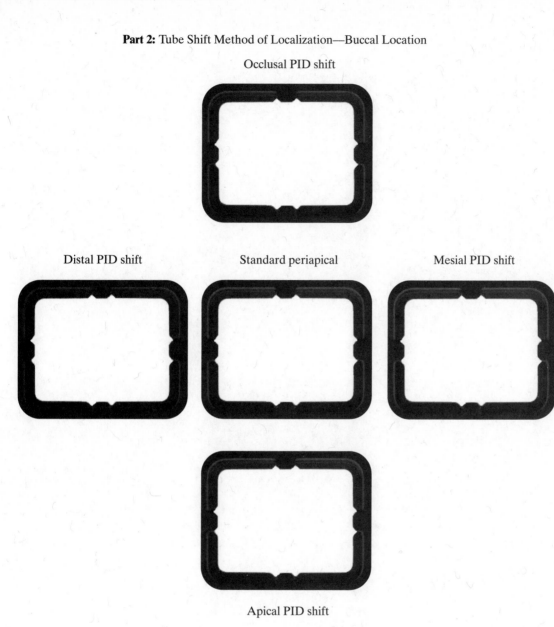

Distal PID shift   Standard periapical   Mesial PID shift

Apical PID shift

Supplemental Radiographic Techniques and Tips   **269**

Part 3: Radiographic Technique Tips for Unique Situations

1. Maxillary molar overlap

2. Canine-first premolar overlap

3. Not recording distal edge of canines

4. Not recording incisal edges

6. Not recording apices

6. Unequal distribution of arches

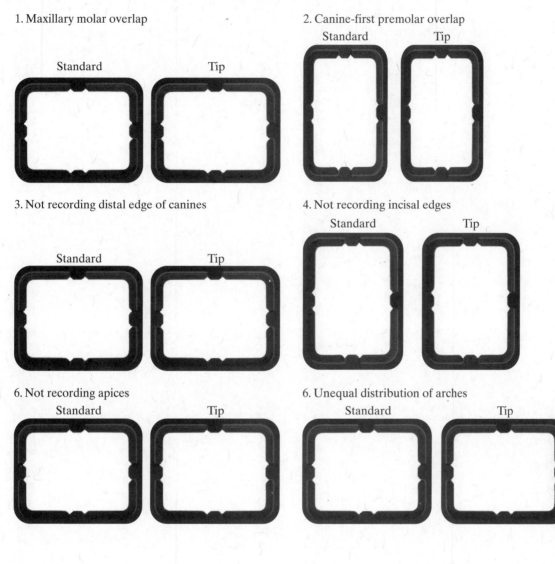

Standard   Tip

Standard   Tip

Standard   Tip

Standard   Tip

Standard   Tip

Standard   Tip

I. Disto-oblique periapical radiographs
  A. Purpose
    1. Record images in the posterior region with minimal discomfort for the patient
    2. May eliminate the need for an extraoral dental radiograph
  B. Uses
    1. Record distally located supernumerary teeth or foreign objects located in the maxillary tuberosity area or the region of the mandibular retromolar pad (Figure 11–14 ■).
    2. Allow imagery in the posterior region of the oral cavity when a patient presents with a hypersensitive gag reflex.
  C. Limitations
    1. Increased image distortion results from an alteration in the vertical angulation.
    2. Increased overlapping of the proximal surfaces results from an alteration in the horizontal angulation.
    3. Image distortion and overlapping are acceptable to achieve the goal of imaging a posteriorly located object (Figure 11–14).
  D. Principal concepts
    1. These radiographs use the same size image receptor as for a standard periapical radiograph.
    2. The horizontal angulation is altered to project the image of the posteriorly located object anteriorly onto the image receptor.
    3. The vertical angulation is altered for the maxillary disto-oblique periapical radiograph to project the apically located object down onto the image receptor.
    4. When using an image receptor holder with an external aiming device such as an arm and ring assembly, the PID and the ring will no longer align with each other (Figure 11–15 ■).

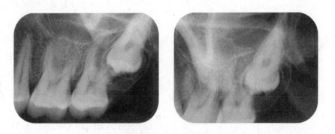

Figure 11–14 A comparison of a standard maxillary molar periapical radiograph (left) and a maxillary disto-oblique periapical radiograph (right). Note the increase in posterior imagery achieved with the disto-oblique periapical radiograph. The increased image distortion and overlap in the disto-oblique periapical radiograph is considered acceptable when utilizing this technique.

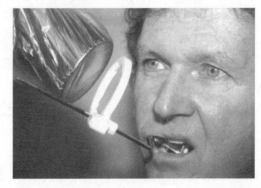

Figure 11–15 Beam alignment for a maxillary disto-oblique periapical radiograph demonstrating how the PID and the external aiming device of the image receptor holder are no longer aligned. Note that altering the horizontal angulation approximately 10 degrees can be estimated by directing the PID approximately 1 to 2 inches away from the aiming ring at an angle that projects the x-rays obliquely toward the image receptor from the distal.

E. Technique—see Table 11-1 Maxillary and Mandibular Disto-oblique Periapical Radiographs
1. The patient is seated upright with the occlusal plane parallel to the floor and the midsagittal plane perpendicular to the floor.
2. Utilizing the paralleling technique, the image receptor is placed as far posteriorly as possible.
3. The horizontal and vertical angulations are first set up as for a standard maxillary posterior periapical radiograph. (See Laboratory Exercise 4, Periapical Radiographs—Paralleling Technique.)
4. From this standard alignment, the PID is then shifted to direct the x-ray beam to project the posterior image onto the image receptor (Figure 11–15).
5. Maxillary disto-oblique periapical radiographs require a change in both the horizontal and vertical angulations and an increased exposure time.
6. Mandibular disto-oblique periapical radiographs require only a change in the horizontal angulation.

II. Localization
A. Purpose
1. Add a third dimension to two-dimensional radiographs
2. Used to determine the buccal or lingual position of an object radiographically
B. Uses
1. Locate the relative position of impactions
2. Identify the location of supernumerary teeth
3. Aid in locating amalgam scrap, broken dental instruments, metallic fragments from accidents
4. Aid endodontic therapy in determining the number and location of root canals
C. Principal concepts
1. These radiographs use the same size image receptor as used for a standard periapical radiograph.
2. The radiographic image of the object of interest is observed following an alteration in the horizontal or vertical angulation of the x-ray beam.
3. Comparing horizontal or vertical beam direction changes with a resulting image shift determines the buccal or lingual position of the object of interest.
D. Methods of localization
1. Right-angle method of localization
a. These radiographs use a cross-sectional occlusal radiograph to determine the buccal-lingual position of an object. (See Laboratory Exercise 10, Occlusal Radiographic Technique.)
b. Once an object has been identified on a standard radiograph, an additional exposure using the cross-sectional occlusal technique is required.
c. These radiographs are more effective on the mandible than the maxilla.
d. This method requires an additional exposure.

2. Tube-shift method of localization
   a. When two objects are in a straight line with the radiographer, one of the objects will be obscured from view.
   b. If the radiographer moves to the right, the more distant object will "move" into view by appearing to shift to the right.
   c. If the radiographer moves to the right, the nearer object will "move" to the left, revealing the more distant object.
   d. Utilizes the buccal-object rule or S.L.O.B. rule
      1) Objects that appear to move in the same direction as the PID shift are located on the lingual—"Same on Lingual."
      2) Objects that appear to move in the opposite direction as the PID shift are located on the buccal—"Opposite on Buccal."
   e. Lingual objects
      1) When the PID shifts to direct the x-ray beam to intersect the image receptor obliquely from the mesial, a lingual object will appear to "move" toward the mesial according to the rule "Same on Lingual."
      2) When the PID shifts to direct the x-ray beam to intersect the image receptor obliquely from the distal, a lingual object will appear to "move" toward the distal according to the rule "Same on Lingual."
      3) When the PID shifts to direct the x-ray beam to intersect the image receptor obliquely from the occlusal, a lingual object will appear to "move" toward the occlusal according to the rule "Same on Lingual."
      4) When the PID shifts to direct the x-ray beam to intersect the image receptor obliquely from the apical, a lingual object will appear to "move" toward the apical according to the rule "Same on Lingual."
   f. Buccal objects
      1) When the PID shifts to direct the x-ray beam to intersect the image receptor obliquely from the mesial, a buccal object will appear to "move" toward the distal according to the rule "Opposite on Buccal."
      2) When the PID shifts to direct the x-ray beam to intersect the image receptor obliquely from the distal, a buccal object will appear to "move" toward the mesial according to the rule "Opposite on Buccal."
      3) When the PID shifts to direct the x-ray beam to intersect the image receptor obliquely from the occlusal, a buccal object will appear to "move" toward the apical according to the rule "Opposite on Buccal."
      4) When the PID shifts to direct the x-ray beam to intersect the image receptor obliquely from the apical, a buccal object will appear to "move" toward the occlusal according to the rule "Opposite on Buccal."
   g. The exposure of an additional radiograph may not be required if the object has been imaged more than once, as in the case of a full mouth or bitewing series of radiographs.

III. Radiographic technique tips
  A. Maxillary molar overlap (Figure 11–16 ■)
    1. Conventional horizontal placement of the image receptor for periapical and bitewing radiographs of the molar region perpendicular to the embrasures of the posterior teeth often results in overlapped contacts between the maxillary first and second molars.
    2. Position the image receptor more perpendicularly to the maxillary first and second molar interproximal space. This is achieved by placing the image receptor diagonally with the anterior portion of the image receptor at a greater distance than the posterior portion from the lingual surfaces of the teeth (Figure 11–8).
  B. Canine-first premolar overlap (Figure 11–17 ■)
    1. Conventional horizontal placement of the image receptor and conventional alignment of the PID for periapical and bitewing radiographs of the canine region often results in overlapping of the contact between the distal portion of the canine with the lingual cusp on the mesial portion of the first premolar.
    2. Angle the image receptor and shift the PID slightly toward the distal to reduce or eliminate the overlap (Figure 11–9).

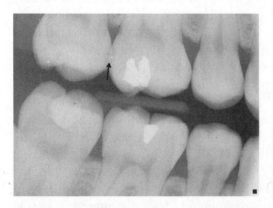

Figure 11–16 Due to the large, rhomboid shape of the maxillary first molars, conventional image receptor placement in this region may still result in overlapped contacts between the maxillary first and second molars.

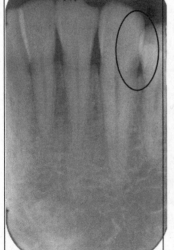
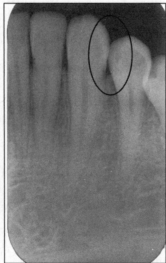

(A)   (B)

Figure 11–17 (A) Conventional image receptor placement and horizontal angulation that results in overlap of the distal portion of the canine with the mesial portion of the lingual cusp of the first premolar. (B) Distal shift in image receptor position and horizontal angulation of the x-ray beam that eliminates overlap of the distal portion of the canine with the mesial portion of the lingual cusp of the first premolar.

C. Not recording the distal edge of the maxillary and mandibular canines on premolar bitewing radiographs
   1. A narrow arch, shallow palate, sensitive lingual mucosa, the presence of tori, or the wire of a digital sensor may hinder positioning the image receptor far enough forward to image the distal portion of both maxillary and mandibular canines.
   2. Angle the image receptor away from the lingual surfaces of the teeth and slide forward to contact the lingual surface of the canine on the opposite side. To avoid overlap error when positioning the image receptor in this manner, the back edge of the image receptor should also be angled slightly away from the lingual surfaces of the teeth. Align the PID to direct the x-rays to intersect the image receptor perpendicularly in this altered position (Figure 11–10).
D. Not recording the incisal/occlusal edges or the apices of the teeth of interest
   1. Excessive vertical angulation results in not recording the incisal/occlusal edges, and inadequate vertical angulation results in not recording the apices of the teeth of interest. Conditions that contribute to incorrect vertical angulation include the manner in which the patient occludes on the biteblock of some image receptor holders, the manner in which a digital sensor in seated into a holding device, and the smaller recording dimensions of digital sensors.
   2. The dental radiographer should have a working knowledge of correct vertical angulation to evaluate the position in the image receptor holding device. If the patient cannot maintain the holder in the correct position, adjust the vertical angulation to the correct position. The external aiming device of the holder should be used as an indicator and not a dictator. Increase or decrease the vertical angulation to the correct position. Allowing the PID to no longer align with the external aiming device is acceptable as long as the increase or decrease is not greater than 15 degrees (Figure 11–11).
   3. If using a digital sensor, assemble into the image receptor holder so that the edge of the sensor will be in position behind the teeth of interest (Figure 11–18 ■).
E. Inadequate distribution of the arches recorded on bitewing radiographs (Figure 11–19 ■)
   1. Long facial cusps of maxillary posterior teeth may force the biteblock of the image receptor into an inadequate vertical angulation position (Figure 11–20 ■).
   2. Increasing the vertical angulation to the correct position, allowing the PID to no longer align with the external aiming device is acceptable as long as the increase is not greater than 15 degrees (Figure 11–21 ■).
   3. Assemble the image receptor holder so that the patient will occlude on the opposite side eliminating excessive contact and the forcing down of the image receptor by the long facial cusps of the maxillary posterior teeth (Figures 11–13 and 11–22 ■).

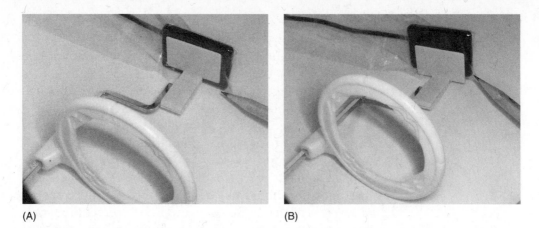

(A)   (B)

Figure 11–18 (A) This assembly of the digital sensor in the image receptor holder may not record the apices of the teeth of interest. (B) Correct assembly to record the entire tooth structures.

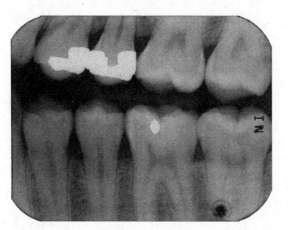

Figure 11–19 Unequal distribution of the arches. Note that less maxillary anatomy is recorded, indicating inadequate vertical angulation.

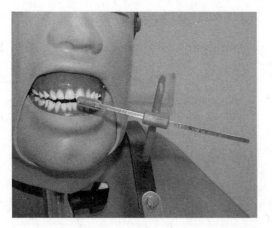

Figure 11–20 Long maxillary facial cusps cause the image receptor holder to be forced down out of correct vertical position.

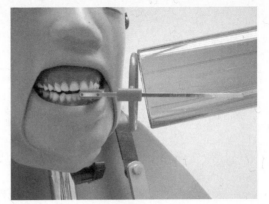

Figure 11–21 Increasing the vertical alignment of the PID to direct the x-rays into the correct vertical angulation.

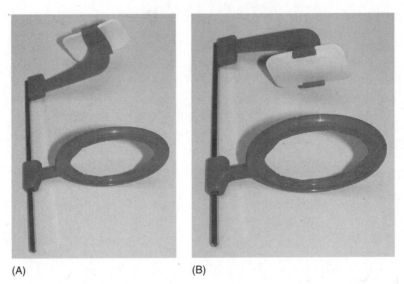

Figure 11–22 (A) Conventional assembly of an image receptor holding device with external arm and aiming ring. (B) Alternate assembly.

(A)   (B)

REFERENCES

O'Carroll, M. K. (1993). *Advanced radiographic techniques part I: Occlusal and lateral oblique projections.* Study guide to videotape series. Chapel Hill, NC: Health Sciences Consortium.

Thomson, E. M., & Johnson, O. N. (2012). *Essentials of dental radiography for dental assistants and hygienists* (9th ed.). Upper Saddle River, NJ: Pearson.

1. Disto-oblique periapical radiographs are indicated for each of the following EXCEPT one. Which one is the EXCEPTION?
   - A. Imaging impacted third molars
   - B. Detection of interproximal caries
   - C. Patient cannot tolerate posterior placement of the image receptor
   - D. Suspected pathology located in the maxillary tuberosity area
   - E. Foreign body suspected in the mandibular retromolar pad region

2. For a maxillary disto-oblique periapical radiograph, the vertical angulation is _____ that used for the standard periapical radiograph.
   - A. increased by 5 degrees over
   - B. decreased by 5 degrees under
   - C. increased by 10 degrees over
   - D. decreased by 10 degrees under

3. For a mandibular disto-oblique periapical radiograph, the horizontal angulation is directed so that x-ray beam will strike the image receptor obliquely
   - A. 5 degrees from the distal.
   - B. 5 degrees from the mesial.
   - C. 10 degrees from the distal.
   - D. 10 degrees from the mesial.

4. For a mandibular disto-oblique periapical radiograph, the exposure setting should be
   - A. increased by one setting over the standard setting.
   - B. decreased by one setting over the standard setting.
   - C. the same as the standard setting.

5. With the tube-shift method of localization, if the PID is shifted to direct the x-ray beam to intersect the image receptor from the mesial, a lingual object will appear to move toward the
   - A. distal.
   - B. mesial.

6. Referring to Part 2: Tube-shift method of localization performed on the maxillary left side of the patient, when the PID shifted to direct the x-ray beam to intersect the image receptor obliquely from the mesial, the object appeared to shift to the
   - A. mesial.
   - B. distal.
   - C. occlusal.
   - D. apical.

7. Referring to Part 2: Tube-shift method of localization performed on the mandibular left side of the patient, when the PID shifted to direct the x-ray beam to intersect the image receptor obliquely from the mesial, the object appeared to shift to the
   A. mesial.
   B. distal.
   C. occlusal.
   D. apical.

8. Which of the following will assist with minimizing molar overlap recorded on a maxillary molar periapical radiograph?
   A. Angle the image receptor toward the lingual surfaces of the teeth and shift the PID slightly toward the distal.
   B. Angle the image receptor away from the lingual surfaces of the teeth and slide forward to contact the canine on the opposite side of the arch.
   C. Angle the posterior edge of the image receptor perpendicular to the first and second molar embrasure.
   D. Angle the anterior edge of the image receptor a greater distance away from the lingual surfaces of the teeth.

9. If an increase in vertical angulation is required to overcome a less than ideal position of the image receptor, an acceptable diagnostic image will result as long as the shift in the vertical angulation is not greater than
   A. 5 degrees.
   B. 10 degrees.
   C. 15 degrees.
   D. 20 degrees.

10. Reversing the biteblock position of a bitewing image receptor holder so that the patient will occlude on the opposite side of the area to be radiographed helps to correct
    A. maxillary molar overlap.
    B. canine-first premolar overlap.
    C. not imaging the apices of the teeth of interest.
    D. imaging an unequal distribution of the arches.

Panoramic Radiographic Technique

INTRODUCTION

There are situations when intraoral radiographs may not provide enough information about a patient's oral condition. The panoramic radiograph is probably the most common extraoral dental radiographic technique. Although not a substitute for an intraoral radiographic examination, the panoramic radiograph plays a valuable role in assessing and diagnosing oral conditions. A panoramic radiograph may be exposed in less time, with minimal patient cooperation, and at a reduced dose of radiation when compared with a full mouth series of intraoral radiographs.

Although panoramic radiography is relatively simple to perform, diagnostic quality depends on precise and exacting steps. While each comes with manufacturer's recommendations for use, there are key steps for exposing panoramic radiographs that are common to most all panoramic x-ray machines. Knowledge of these key points not only will allow the dental radiographer to produce quality radiographic images with any machine, but also will aid in applying corrective measures to less than ideal imagery.

The purpose of this laboratory exercise is to introduce the basic steps required for panoramic radiography and to provide an opportunity to practice the procedure. Not all panoramic x-ray machines operate exactly the same, however, achieving a quality panoramic radiograph depends on a working knowledge of six key steps: (1) cassette and film or photostimuable phosphor PSP plate preparation and care, (2) unit preparation, (3) patient preparation, (4) patient positioning, (5) exposure, and (6) processing (film-based images) and scanning (PSP plates). Together, with a student partner, you will simulate preparing a panoramic image receptor and readying the panoramic x-ray machine for exposure. Patient preparation and positioning will be practiced on each other, establishing a real-life setting in which to become familiar with the operation of the panoramic equipment. *WARNING:* DO NOT ACTIVATE THE EXPOSURE BUTTON. DO NOT EXPOSE YOUR STUDENT PARTNER TO RADIATION. YOU ARE PRACTICING PATIENT PREPARATION AND POSITIONING ONLY. YOU WILL NOT ACTUALLY EXPOSE A PRACTICE RADIOGRAPH.

OBJECTIVES

Following completion of this lab activity, you will be able to:

1. Demonstrate proficiency in preparing the panoramic image receptor for exposure.

2. Demonstrate correct patient positioning to achieve a quality panoramic radiograph.

3. Identify and apply corrective actions for common image receptor care and handling, unit preparation, patient preparation and positioning, exposure, and processing errors that compromise the quality of a panoramic radiograph.

MATERIALS

Panoramic x-ray machine (film-based, photostimuable phosphor (PSP) plate, or direct digital technology)

Panoramic cassette with intensifying screens and practice film or PSP plate

Student partner

Lead/lead equivalent cape or apron with no thyroid collar attached

Handwashing station with antimicrobial soap or antiseptic hand rub

Disinfectant

Paper towels

Heavy duty utility gloves

PREPARATION

1. Study the chapter outline to prepare for this laboratory exercise. An understanding of the material presented in the outline is required to complete this activity.

2. Together with a student partner, use the panoramic procedure evaluation to assess your ability to satisfactorily perform each of the steps of the panoramic radiographic procedure.
   WARNING: DO NOT ACTIVATE THE EXPOSURE BUTTON. DO NOT EXPOSE YOUR STUDENT PARTNER TO RADIATION. YOU ARE PRACTICING THESE SKILLS. YOU WILL NOT ACTUALLY EXPOSE A RADIOGRAPH.

3. Instructor demonstration may enhance knowledge of the laboratory exercise.

4. Obtain instructor feedback on your performance as necessary or as instructed.

LABORATORY EXERCISE ACTIVITIES

Part 1: Cassette and Image Receptor Preparation

1. Obtain cassette with intensifying screens and a practice film or cassette without intensifying screens and photostimuable phosphor (PSP) plate.

Direct digital panoramic machines have a build-in sensor. A cassette is not required.

2. Use Procedure 12–1 to practice cassette and image receptor preparation.

3. Designate an area with counter space for this activity. Realistically, this preparation step would be performed in the darkroom. However, practicing this step with the lights on may help you visualize the skills you are developing.

Part 2: Unit Preparation

Together with a student partner, use Procedure 12–1 to prepare the panoramic radiographic machine and image receptor. Follow infection control protocol.

Part 3: Patient Preparation

With your student partner playing the role of the patient, proceed with the steps outlined in Procedure 12–1 to prepare your patient for the panoramic radiograph.

Part 4: Patient Positioning

Position your student partner into the panoramic unit following the guidelines outlined in Procedure 12–1. Note that the patient must be positioned into all three dimensions of the focal trough.

Part 5: Exposure

1. Select appropriate exposure setting and simulate exposure.
   WARNING: REMEMBER THAT YOU ARE PRACTICING PANORAMIC POSITIONING ONLY. DO NOT EXPOSE YOUR STUDENT PARTNER TO RADIATION.

2. Utilize guidelines outlined in Procedure 12–1.

3. Release the patient.

4. Perform infection control protocol following the procedure.

COMPETENCY AND EVALUATION

1. Switch student partner roles and repeat this exercise. The student patient should now play the role of radiographer, and the student radiographer should now play the role of patient, so that both partners have the opportunity to complete this exercise.

2. When both you and your partner have completed the exercise, each of you should review the panoramic procedure evaluation (Procedure 12–1) and determine what skills you found the most challenging and/or the easiest to learn.

What steps do you anticipate being the easiest to master? Why?

What steps do you anticipate being the most difficult to achieve? Why?

What are some examples of directions you had to give to the patient to achieve his or her cooperation with the procedure?

What visual guides did the manufacturer of the panoramic machine provide you for positioning the patient correctly? Explain how you used these guides to position the patient within the focal trough.

3. Complete the study questions.

Procedure 12–1

Panoramic Procedure Evaluation

Cassette and Image Receptor Preparation

Film-based:

1. Examine the cassette for proper function. _____

    a. Examine the cassette for warping (rigid cassettes) or tears (plastic sleeve cassettes). _____

    b. Check the hinge or Velcro® seal for secure closing and a light-tight seal (see Figure 13–9). _____

2. Examine the intensifying screens for quality. _____

    a. Check for scratches. _____

    b. Check for need of cleaning. Clean only as necessary and as recommended by manufacturer. (Aggressive cleaning can damage screens.) Apply a manufacturer-recommended antistatic solution as necessary. _____

3. Ensure that the intensifying screens are properly secured to the cassette (rigid cassette) or are properly loaded into the flexible cassette. (Screens should be folded with the printed information identifying the screen manufacturer and screen type on the inside of the fold.) (Figure 12–1 ■) _____

4. Obtain a box of panoramic film and place the film box and cassette with intensifying screens on darkroom counter. Turn off the white overhead light and turn on the safelight. _____

5. Open the box of panoramic film, remove one sheet of panoramic film, and place in the cassette between the intensifying screens. Close the cassette and hinge to ensure a light-tight position. Resecure the panoramic film box and return to its storage place. _____

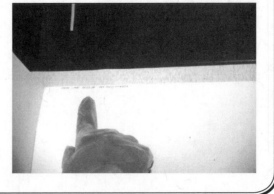

Figure 12–1 The side of the intensifying screens with the manufacturer's labeling should be facing the film.

(continued)

Procedure 12–1 (continued)

Photostimuable phosphor (PSP) plate technology:

1. Examine the cassette for proper function. _____

   a. Examine the cassette for warping (rigid cassettes) or tears (plastic sleeve cassettes). _____

   b. Check the hinge or Velcro® seal for secure closing and a light-tight seal (see Figure 13–9). _____

2. Insert the PSP plate into the cassette. Be sure that the correct side faces the radiation source. Intensifying screens are not required for PSP exposures. _____

Digital sensor technology:

1. The digital sensor is built in to the panoramic machine. Cassette and intensifying screens are not required (Figure 12–2 ■). _____

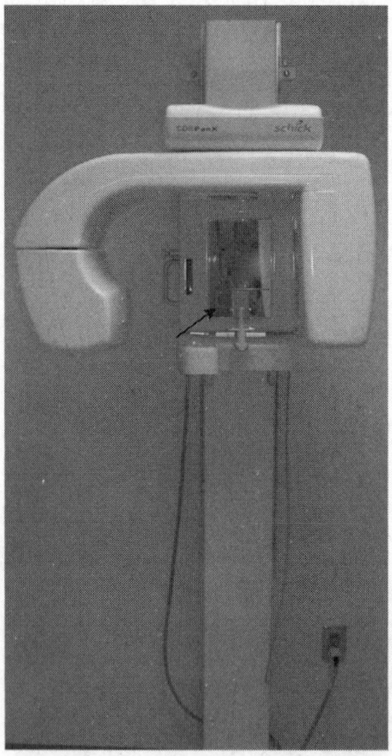

Figure 12–2 Digital panoramic x-ray machine with sensor build into rotational arm. Note the mirror that will be used as an aid to position the patient's arches within the focal trough.

(continued)

Procedure 12-1 (continued)

Unit Preparation

1. Clean and disinfect and cover with an appropriate barrier all surfaces that will contact the patient either directly or indirectly. See the following list (Figure 12–3 ■):

   a. Chin rest   _____

   b. Head positioner guides   _____

   c. Support handles   _____

   d. Chair or seat (sit down units only)   _____

   e. Lead/lead equivalent cape or apron without a thyroid collar   _____

2. Select a sterile (disposable or autoclavable) bite guide. Load into the bite guide holder. (Use a sterile cotton roll to separate the arches if a bite guide is not used by the unit manufacturer.)   _____

3. Attach the cassette with film or PSP plate to the panoramic x-ray machine according to the manufacturer's instructions. Align the cassette into proper position using guidelines established by manufacturer (Figure 12–4 ■).   _____

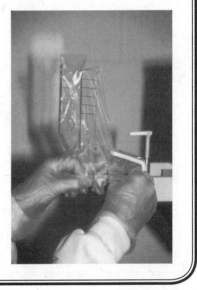

Figure 12–3 Plastic barriers may be placed over the chin rest, head positioner guides, and other parts of the panoramic unit that contact the patient.

(continued)

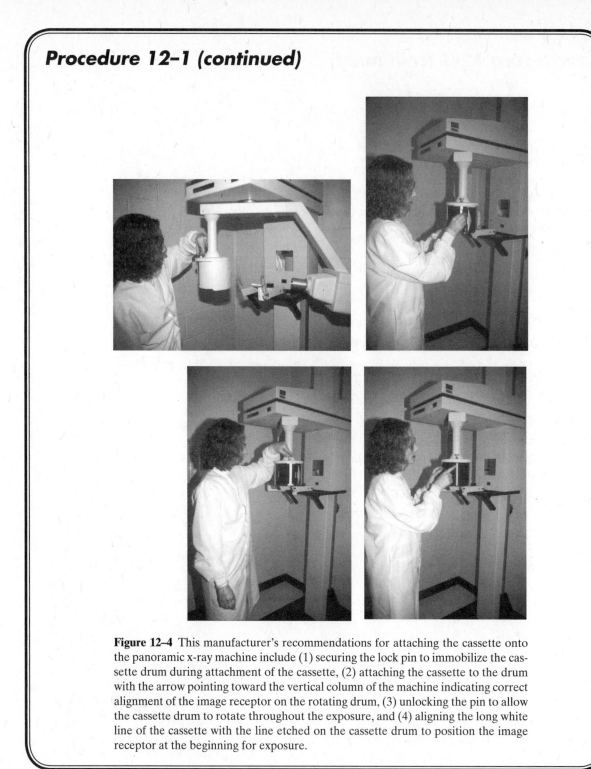

Figure 12–4 This manufacturer's recommendations for attaching the cassette onto the panoramic x-ray machine include (1) securing the lock pin to immobilize the cassette drum during attachment of the cassette, (2) attaching the cassette to the drum with the arrow pointing toward the vertical column of the machine indicating correct alignment of the image receptor on the rotating drum, (3) unlocking the pin to allow the cassette drum to rotate throughout the exposure, and (4) aligning the long white line of the cassette with the line etched on the cassette drum to position the image receptor at the beginning for exposure.

(continued)

Procedure 12-1 (continued)

Patient Preparation

1. Assess the patient for need of panoramic survey.   _____

2. Inform the patient of the need for the radiograph, explain the   _____
   procedure and rationale, answer patient concerns/questions regarding
   the radiographic procedure, and obtain the patient's written consent.

3. Request that the patient remove eyeglasses, necklaces, hair barrettes,   _____
   facial jewelry (tongue, lip piercing adornments), removable dental
   appliances, and any other material that may interfere with the
   radiographic procedure such as chewing gum or a hooded sweatshirt
   that is bulky in the neck region.

4. Place the lead/lead equivalent cape or apron without a lead thyroid   _____
   collar over the patient (Figure 12–5 ■).

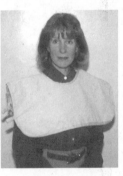

Figure 12–5 Cape-style lead/lead equivalent barrier without a thyroid collar, appropriate for protecting the patient during exposure of a panoramic radiograph.

*Satisfactorily
Performed*
✓

Patient Positioning

1. To position the patient into the focal trough's anterior/posterior   _____
   dimension, instruct him or her to bite on the bite guide with the anterior
   teeth occluding edge-to-edge, or to place the chin completely forward into
   the chin rest, or to place the forehead against the forehead rest
   (Figure 12–6 ■). Use the panoramic machine's indictor light, if so equipped,
   to locate the correct anterior/posterior position (Figure 12–7 ■).

2. To position the patient into the focal trough's lateral (right/left)   _____
   dimension, close the head positioner guides, or instruct the patient
   to view his or her reflection in the mirror (if available) and align the
   midsagittal plane perpendicular to the floor (Figures 12–2 and 12–8 ■).
   Use the panoramic machine's indictor light, if so equipped, to locate
   the midsagittal plane (Figure 12–7).

(continued)

Procedure 12–1 (continued)

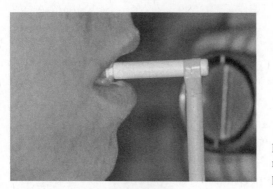

Figure 12–6 The bite guide of this panoramic x-ray machine is used to place the patient's arches into the proper anterior/posterior position within the focal trough.

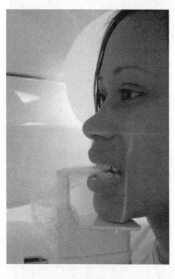

Figure 12–7 This panoramic x-ray machine uses laser light guides to assist with placing the patient's arches into the proper position within the focal trough.

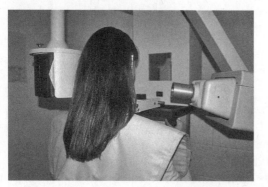

Figure 12–8 The mirror and head positioner guides of this panoramic unit are used to place the patient's arches into the proper lateral position within the focal trough.

3. To position the patient into the focal trough's superior/inferior dimension, _____ adjust the patient's chin up or down until the Frankfort plane is parallel to the floor or the ala-tragus line is tipped down 5 degrees. Some panoramic x-ray machines have indicator lines scribed on the head positioner guides or projected as a beam of light from the unit to align either the Frankfort plane or the ala-tragus line to obtain correct superior/inferior patient positioning in the focal trough (Figures 12–7 and 12–9 ■).

(continued)

Procedure 12–1 (continued)

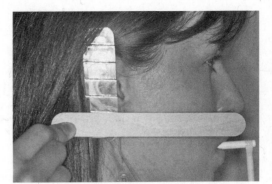

Figure 12–9 This panoramic x-ray unit utilizes scribed lines on the head positioner guides to aid in aligning the ala-tragus line 5 degrees with the floor. (*Note:* A tongue blade may be used as a guide to achieving correct alignment.)

Satisfactorily
Performed
✓

4. Direct the patient to close the lips around the bite guide or a cotton roll to prevent imaging the soft tissue shadow of the lip line.   _____

5. Direct the patient to swallow and place the tongue against the roof of the mouth and hold it there throughout the exposure cycle to fill in the oral cavity and to minimize the appearance of a large radiolucent image of an open air space.   _____

6. Instruct the patient to remain still throughout the exposure cycle.   _____

Exposure

1. Select the appropriate kVp and mA for this patient. Refer to posted exposure settings (Figure 12–10 ■). The exposure time setting is preset by the manufacturer.   _____

2. Take an appropriate position where you are protected from radiation exposure and simulate depressing the exposure button for the duration of the cycle.   _____

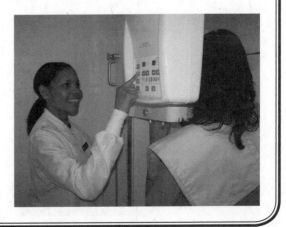
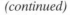

Figure 12–10 Radiographer selects the appropriate exposure settings.

(continued)

Procedure 12–1 (continued)

3. Release the patient. Remove barriers and discard the disposable bite guide or, if autoclavable, prepare for sterilization. Clean and disinfect with appropriate disinfectant all surfaces that came in contact, either directly or indirectly, with the patient. See the following list:

   a. Chin rest _____

   b. Head positioner guides _____

   c. Support handles _____

   d. Chair or seat (sit down units only) _____

   e. Lead/lead equivalent cape or apron without a thyroid collar _____

Satisfactorily
Performed
✓

Processing

Film-based:

1. Remove the cassette with film from the panoramic rotational arm, and return to the darkroom. Turn off the overhead white light, and turn on the safe light. _____

2. Open the cassette and carefully remove the film. Handle with clean dry, ungloved hands. Load the film into the automatic processor or the manual film processing rack for processing. _____

3. Label the processed film with the patient's name, date, and other pertinent information.* _____

*NOTE: If using a commercial flash identification printer, complete the printer card with the patient's name, date of birth, and name of the practice setting, and flash print after the exposure, but prior to processing the film (Figure 12–11 ■).

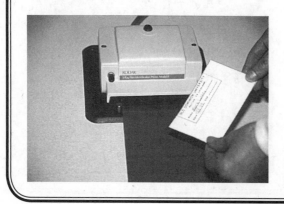

Figure 12–11 A flash printer may be used to identify a radiographic film.

(continued)

Procedure 12–1 (continued)

Satisfactorily Performed ✓

Photostimuable phosphor (PSP) plate technology:

1. Remove the cassette with PSP plate from the panoramic rotational arm and proceed to the location of the laser scanner and computer. _____
2. Open the cassette and carefully remove the PSP plate. Handle with clean dry, ungloved hands. Load into the laser scanner and activate. _____
3. Observe the image on the computer monitor. _____

Digital sensor technology:

1. Digital sensor is built into the panoramic machine and will capture and display the image almost immediately on the computer monitor (Figure 12–12 ■). _____

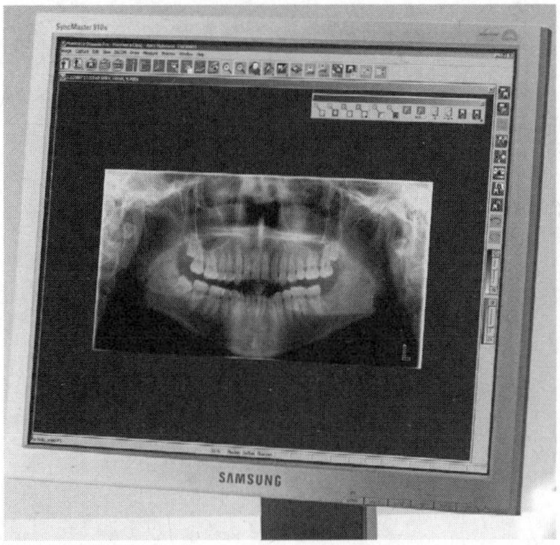

Figure 12–12 A panoramic digital image displayed on the computer monitor. (Courtesy of Planmeca)

I. Panoramic radiography
   A. Uses
      1. Detection of large lesions
      2. Evaluation of unexplained asymmetry
      3. Assessing growth and development
      4. Assessing the need for orthodontic intervention
      5. Detection of fractures in supporting bone
      6. Evaluation of third molar impactions
      7. Assessment of condition of underlying bone prior to implants or denture construction
   B. Advantages over intraoral radiographs
      1. Increased coverage of supporting structures of the oral cavity
      2. Reduced patient radiation dose over an intraoral full mouth series of radiographs
      3. Can be performed in less time than the exposure of a full mouth series of radiographs
      4. Simple procedure to perform
      5. Not necessary for the patient to tolerate intraoral placement of image receptor
      6. May be performed on patients who cannot tolerate placement of an image receptor
      7. Requires minimal patient instruction and cooperation
      8. Infection control protocol minimized
      9. Panoramic broad-view image of the entire arches is easy for patients to understand when utilizing for patient education and in explaining treatment plans
   C. Limitations
      1. Image distortion is increased.
      2. Image sharpness is reduced.
      3. Focal trough size and shape limits recording only those structures that fit into the image layer.
      4. Soft tissue shadows and ghost images present on the resulting image may hinder interpretation.
      5. It is not useful in detecting incipient carious lesions or early periodontal changes.
      6. Simple procedure may cause the panoramic radiograph to be overused inappropriately as a screening for occult disease.
      7. Length of exposure time may limit its use on young children and other patients who cannot remain still throughout the exposure cycle.
      8. The cost of a panoramic unit may be a significant burden on the practice.
   D. Overview of equipment fundamentals
      1. Intensifying screens
         a. These screens convert x-ray energy into visible light, "intensifying" the effect of x-rays on film.
         b. Radiation exposure can be reduced because this fluorescent light aids in the production of the image.
         c. Screens are paired and attached or sandwiched into a cassette.

2. Cassette
   a. May be rigid or flexible
   b. Must be attached to panoramic x-ray machine according to manufacturer's recommendations so that the image receptor will be aligned to move in the appropriate direction once the cycle begins
3. Image receptors
   a. Panoramic film type must match the type of intensifying screens.
      1) Rare earth intensifying screens fluoresce green light and must be paired with extraoral film that is sensitive to green light.
      2) Calcium tungstate intensifying screens fluoresce blue light and must be paired with extraoral film that is sensitive to blue light.
   b. Photostimuable phosphor (PSP) plate technology does not require the use of intensifying screens.
      1) PSP technology uses a polyester plate coated with a storage phosphor (europium activated barium fluorohalide) that captures the image in a manner similar to silver halide crystals within film emulsion.
      2) After exposure, the PSP plate is placed into a laser scanner that sends a signal to a computer.
      3) The computer uses the data contained in the digital signal to reconstruct an image on a computer monitor.
   c. Direct digital panoramic x-ray machines have a built-in solid-state sensor that captures the x-radiation.
      1) The sensor is attached to the rotational arm of the panoramic x-ray machine in the same location as the film drum, allowing it to rotate in relation to the rotating tube head and x-ray source.
      2) The computer uses the data contained in the digital signal to reconstruct an image on a computer monitor.
4. Rotational x-ray tube head
   a. The tube head has a fixed vertical angulation of the PID at approximately negative 8 degrees.
   b. Collimation of the PID produces a narrow, fan shaped x-ray beam (Figure 12–13 ■).
5. Cassette holder (drum)

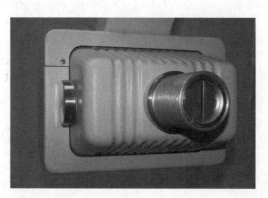

Figure 12–13 Panoramic x-ray machine PID (position indicating device) is collimated to produce a narrow, fan-shaped x-ray beam.

a. The cassette used for film-based and phosphor plate panoramic x-ray machines attaches to the cassette holder. Direct digital panoramic x-ray machines have a built-in sensor in the place where a cassette holder would be located (Figure 12–2).

b. The cassette holder moves the image receptor at the same speed as the rotational x-ray beam.

6. Patient positioning guides

a. Anterior/posterior position is determined through the use of a bite guide, forehead rest, or anterior edge of the chin rest. Some panoramic machines are equipped with a light beam that when activated, shines on the patient's face to assist with determining the correct anterior/posterior position.

b. Lateral (right/left) position is determined through the use of side head positioner guides, a mirror, or beams of light that shine on the patient's face to assist with determining the position of the midsagittal plane.

c. Superior/inferior position is determined through the use of a chin rest or beams of light that shine on the patient's face to assist with determining the position of the Frankfort plane or ala-tragus line.

7. Exposure control panel (Figure 12–14 ■)

a. Variable kVp

1) Setting is recommended by manufacturer.

2) kVp setting is usually based on the size and density of the patient and the area to be imaged.

b. Variable or fixed mA

c. Fixed exposure time

1) Preset by the manufacturer

2) Approximately 15–20 seconds to complete the exposure cycle

E. Technique

1. Based on the principle of tomography

a. A "slice" or "layer" of tissue is imaged.

b. Several different x-ray beam movement patterns are utilized to produce an image.

c. Each section of the simultaneously moving image receptor is exposed until the entire image is complete.

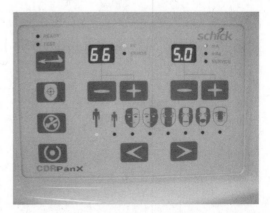

Figure 12–14 Digital panoramic x-ray machine control panel with variable settings.

2. Focal trough
   a. This is a horseshoe-shaped area corresponding to the shape of the average dental arches.
      1) Focal trough size and shape are determined by the manufacturer.
      2) Average dimensions do not always accommodate every patient.
      3) Some units have multiple focal trough sizes to accommodate adult and child patients
   b. Objects located in the focal trough will be imaged in acceptable detail on the resultant radiograph.
   c. Objects located outside the focal trough will be blurred out of focus on the resultant radiograph.
      1) Creates ghost images that may compromise image clarity.
      2) Objects positioned outside the focal trough may not be detected.

F. Labeling
   1. Most panoramic x-ray machines have a method of indicating left and right sides of the radiograph (Figure 12–15 ■).
   2. If the panoramic x-ray machine does not have a built-in method of labeling the right and left sides of the radiograph, a lead/metal letter may be affixed to the cassette prior to exposing.
   3. Radiographic tape is also available to label panoramic radiographs with patient name and other identifying characteristics (Figure 12–16 ■).

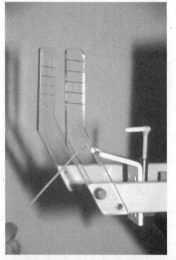

Figure 12–15 A lead/metal letter is used by this panoramic x-ray machine to identify the right side of the patient's radiograph.

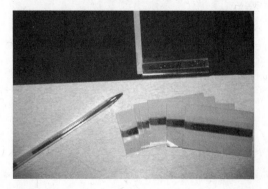

Figure 12–16 Radiographic tape may be used to identify a film-based panoramic radiograph.

4. A commercial flash printer machine permanently records pertinent information onto the radiograph (Figure 12–11).

II. Identification of panoramic errors
   A. Cassette and image receptor preparation errors
      1. Cassette not closed light tight. Evidenced by an increased density from accidental light exposure.
      2. Film not seated at the fold of (flexible plastic-sleeve) cassette. Evidenced by a portion of the radiograph not exposed (blank/clear).
      3. Intensifying screens placed into the cassette inside out (with manufacturer's labeling on the outside) (Figure 12–1). Evidenced by an overall blank/clear or very light image.
      4. Film not placed in between the intensifying screens (flexible plastic-sleeve cassette). Evidenced by an overall blank/clear or very light image.
      5. Mistaken use of duplicating film instead of panoramic film (Figure 12–17 ■). Evidenced by a blank/clear radiograph because duplicating film is not responsive to x-radiation exposure.
      6. Intensifying screens scratched or damaged. Evidenced by radiopaque artifacts corresponding to the damaged screen area.
      7. Double exposure. Evidenced by a dark image of two separate exposures superimposed on top of each other.
      8. Bright light exposure (photostimuable phosphor [PSP] plate). Evidenced by a blank/clear or very light image as the PSP plates are erased by bright light exposure.
   B. Unit preparation errors
      1. Cassette drum (film-based and photostimuable phosphor [PSP] plate) not set to rotate freely throughout the exposure. Evidenced by a blank/clear image with a dense vertical band of overexposure, representing the only area of the image receptor to be exposed.
      2. Cassette (film-based and photostimuable phosphor [PSP] plate) not correctly aligned to begin exposure at the beginning of the cycle. Evidenced by a generally blank/clear image with a narrow band of exposure at one end, representing where the image receptor proceeded to rotate in the opposite direction of the radiation source.
   C. Patient preparation errors
      1. Tube head or cassette holder (drum) contacted the patient's shoulder during rotation. Evidenced by radiolucent vertical

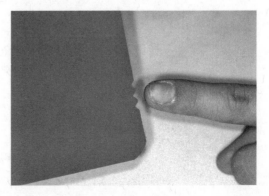

Figure 12–17 Duplicating film is distinguished from panoramic film by the notched edge placed by the manufacturer.

Panoramic Radiographic Technique

band(s) of overexposure in the areas where the rotational arm of the machine was stopped temporarily, overexposing certain regions of the image receptor.

2. Patient wore a metal or dense object that was in the path of the x-ray beam during exposure. Evidenced by radiopaque artifacts from the object left in the path of the x-ray beam; artifacts of the object's ghost image will most likely be evident on the opposite side of the image.

3. A lead/lead equivalent thyroid collar was used during the exposure. Evidenced by an unexposed area, usually located at the inferior edge of the radiograph where the collar blocked the radiation.

D. Patient positioning errors

1. Arches not positioned in the anterior/posterior dimension of the focal trough. Evidenced by the appearance of narrowed anterior teeth indicating the arches were positioned too far anterior in the focal trough or widened anterior teeth indicating that the arches were positioned too far posterior in the focal trough.

2. Arches not positioned in the lateral (right/left) dimension of the focal trough. Evidenced by narrowed and severely overlapped posterior teeth on the side to which the arches were turned or tilted toward, and widened and magnified posterior teeth on the other side from which the arches were turned or tilted away from.

3. Arches not positioned in the superior/inferior dimension of the focal trough. Evidenced by an exaggerated "frown" appearance to the overall image when the arches are positioned too far superior in the focal trough (chin up) and by an exaggerated "smile" appearance to the overall image when the arches are positioned too far inferior in the focal trough (chin down).

4. Patient not standing/sitting up straight. Evidenced by a radiopaque ghost image of the compressed cervical vertebrae of the spinal column usually superimposed over the mandibular anterior teeth.

5. Lips not closed around the biteblock. Evidenced by an image of the soft tissue shadow of the lip line superimposed across the anterior teeth that can mimic the appearance of caries or a tooth fracture.

6. Tongue not placed flat against the palate during exposure. Evidenced by a large radiolucency superimposed over the maxillary teeth apices.

E. Exposure errors

1. Incorrect exposure setting selected. Evidenced by an over/underexposed image.

2. Bite guide or cotton roll not utilized to separate the arches. Evidenced by incisal/occlusal edges of the maxillary and mandibular teeth superimposed on top of each other.

3. Patient moved during the procedure. Evidenced by a blurred portion or irregular margins of the image.

F. Processing errors

1. Over/underdeveloped. Evidenced by an image that is too dark/light.

2. Static electricity artifacts. Evidenced by radiolucent lines, spots, or smudges indicating white light exposure from the static charge.
3. Glove powder artifacts. Evidenced by radiolucent powder smudges.

REFERENCES

Eastman Kodak. (2000). *Successful panoramic radiography.* Rochester, NY: Author.

Horner, K., Drage, N., & Brettle, D. (2008). *21st Century Imaging.* London: Quintessence Publishing Co., Ltd.

Rushton, V. E., & Rout, J. (2006). *Panoramic radiography.* London: Quintessence Publishing Co., Ltd.

Serman, N., Horrell, B. M., & Singer, S. (2003). High-quality panoramic radiographs. Tips and tricks. *Dent Today, 22*(1), 70–3.

Thomson, E. M. (2009). Focusing on the image. How to produce error-free radiographic images for the pediatric patient. *Dimen Dent Hyg, 7*(2), 24–26, 27.

Thomson, E. M., & Johnson, O. N. (2012). *Essentials of dental radiography for dental assistants and hygienists* (9th ed.). Upper Saddle River, NJ: Pearson.

1. Each of the following is an indication for exposing a panoramic radiograph EXCEPT one. Which one is the EXCEPTION?
   - A. Caries detection
   - B. Location of an impaction
   - C. Evaluation of eruption patterns
   - D. Imaging a large lesion

2. Which of the following is NOT true regarding panoramic radiographs?
   - A. Can be performed in less time than the exposure of a full mouth series of radiographs imaging
   - B. Provide an acceptable image for patient who cannot tolerate placement of an intraoral image receptor
   - C. Require minimal patient cooperation and is easy to tolerate
   - D. Require more radiation than exposure of a full mouth series of intraoral radiographs

3. What is the role of intensifying screens?
   - A. Provide a light-tight holder for panoramic extraoral film
   - B. Send a digital signal of the image that can be read by a computer
   - C. Convert x-ray energy into visible light
   - D. Capture the image in a manner similar to silver halide crystals within film emulsion

4. Which of the following terms refers to the horseshoe-shaped zone of sharpness where an object will be imaged in acceptable detail?
   - A. Cassette drum
   - B. Ghost image
   - C. Intensifying screen
   - D. Focal trough

5. Which of the following is NOT a dimension of the focal trough?
   - A. Anterior-posterior
   - B. Parallel-perpendicular
   - C. Superior-inferior
   - D. Left-right

6. When a patient's arches are positioned too far to the right, the teeth on the _____ side of the image will appear narrowed and severely overlapped.
   - A. right
   - B. left

7. When a patient's arches are positioned too far forward in the focal trough, the anterior teeth will appear
   - A. widened.
   - B. narrowed

8. What panoramic patient positioning error will result in dental arches that appear as an exaggerated smile?
   A. Patient was not standing up straight.
   B. Patient did not close lips around the biteblock.
   C. Patient's chin was tilted up too high.
   D. Patient's chin was tilted down too low.

9. A dark shadow obscuring the apices of the maxillary anterior teeth is most likely caused by which of the following?
   A. Lead/lead equivalent thyroid collar got in the way
   B. Facial jewelry not removed
   C. Chin not in position against chin rest
   D. Tongue not resting against palate
   E. Teeth not occluded on bite guide/cotton roll

10. A patient who wears a maxillary full denture needs a panoramic radiograph. All of his natural mandibular teeth are in place. You will request that the patient remove the denture during the exposure. What patient positioning step do you anticipate having the most difficulty achieving? If an error is made in this step, how will the resultant image look? Why? What corrective actions would you take? Why?

_____

_____

_____

_____

_____

_____

_____

_____

_____

_____

Radiographic Quality Assurance

INTRODUCTION

Dental radiographic quality increases when a carefully administered quality assurance program is in place. Ensuring the production of diagnostic quality radiographs while also minimizing radiation exposure is the definition of quality assurance. To be effective, quality assurance requires a plan of action. This plan is referred to as quality control. Quality control is the means of testing and regulating x-ray equipment and procedures used to expose, process, and store radiographic images. The benefits of quality control include improved patient care through production of quality radiographic images, decreased radiation exposure because retake radiographs are avoided, and time and monetary savings both for the patient and for the oral health care practice. The time spent developing and implementing a quality assurance program is worth the benefits gained.

X-ray equipment is regulated by federal, state, and local regulations, which usually include inspections and evaluation of equipment, but the radiographer plays an important role in the daily monitoring of equipment. It may be convenient to assign equipment testing to these expert inspectors. However, the dental radiographer is ultimately responsible for the equipment at the time of use. The dental radiographer should possess a working knowledge of the equipment utilized and understand when results produced by this equipment are below standard.

The purpose of this exercise is to introduce several quality control tests that the radiographer can use to periodically monitor equipment and procedures. Performing the quality control tests in this exercise provides a twofold benefit. First, you will gain experience in evaluating the performance of radiographic equipment, and second, the results of your activities may help fulfill the quality assurance required on your institution's equipment.

OBJECTIVES

Following completion of this lab activity, you will be able to:

1. Identify the role the radiographer plays in establishing and maintaining a quality assurance program.

2. Perform quality control tests on the equipment used to process dental radiographs.

3. Perform quality control tests to monitor stored dental radiographic film.

4. Perform quality control tests on the equipment used to expose dental radiographs.

5. Value establishing a quality assurance program for the oral health care practice.

MATERIALS

Size #2 radiographic films

Size #2 photostimuable phosphor (PSP) plates

Sample pre-fogged film

Step-wedge (commercially made or made from discarded lead foils using Procedure 13–1)

Coin (such as a penny)

Three different metal identification items (paper clip, tack, safety pin, etc.)

Viewbox

PREPARATION

1. Study the chapter outline to prepare for this laboratory exercise. An understanding of the material presented in the outline is required to complete this activity.

2. Designate an area, countertop, or operatory chair for this exercise.

3. Instructor demonstration may enhance knowledge of the laboratory exercise.

Procedure 13–1

Instructions for Assembling a Step Wedge (Figure 13–1 ■)

Varying the thickness or density of an object can vary the amount of radiation reaching the image receptor. A step wedge is constructed of a radiopaque material arranged to vary in thickness from decreased density to increased density. Follow these instructions to assemble a step wedge to use in the following quality control tests. Compare your step wedge with the one pictured in Figure 13–2 ■.

1. Obtain six sheets of lead foil from intraoral film packets.
2. Assemble three piles of two lead foil sheets each.
3. Layer each of the three piles into "steps" of increasing thickness
4. Tape securely together.

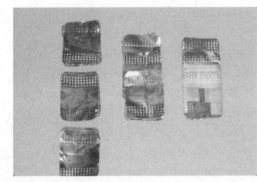

Figure 13–1 (Left) Six sheets of lead foil assembled into three piles of two sheets each. (Middle) Each of the three piles have been layered into "steps" of increasing thickness. (Right) Finished step wedge secured with tape.

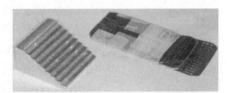

Figure 13–2 (Left) A commercially made step wedge. (Right) A step wedge assembled from intraoral film packet lead foil sheets.

Part 1: Quality Control Test for Effectiveness of Processing Chemistry—Reference Film

The purpose of this activity is to monitor the daily strength of the processing chemistry. Manufacturers recommend replenishing and completely changing processing solutions at preset intervals, but actual usage may dictate that solutions be changed more or less frequently than these recommendations. Ideally, solutions should be tested for optimal processing strength daily, or twice daily in the case of extremely high usage as occurs in a clinical setting. Solutions should be changed prior to reducing the quality of a patient's radiographs.

1. Obtain two size #2 radiographic film packets.
2. Check posted exposure settings for the dental x-ray machine and set for the maxillary central incisor periapical radiograph.
3. Prepare to expose the first film by placing it tube side up on the countertop or operatory chair.
4. Place the step-wedge on top of the film packet.
5. Direct the PID (position indicating device) over the film packet and step-wedge. Maintain a distance of 1 inch between the edge of the PID and the film packet and step-wedge (Figure 13–3 ■).
6. Expose the first film and step-wedge. Set aside.
7. Immediately expose the second film and step-wedge using the same x-ray machine, at the same settings, in the same manner.
8. Assuming it is the beginning of your laboratory session and that the processing chemicals are fresh, process one of the exposed films now. Set the other exposed film aside to be processed at the end of the laboratory session.
9. Continue with the rest of the exercise. At the end of the laboratory session, process the film you exposed and set aside at the beginning of the laboratory session.

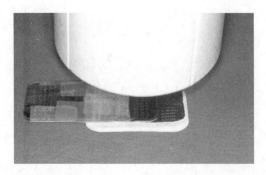

Figure 13–3 Assembled step wedge and film packet image receptor ready for exposure. Note that the PID is in position approximately 1 inch above the image receptor-step wedge combination.

Part 2: Quality Control Test for Adequacy of Darkroom Safelighting—Coin Test

The purpose of this activity is to evaluate the adequacy of the safelighting conditions in the darkroom. This test is most valuable when performed as a true simulation. Because film that has been exposed, as is the case with patient films, is more sensitive to exposure by white light, you will be pre-exposing the films before performing the coin test. Additionally, allowing your test film to remain opened on the darkroom counter for 2 minutes will simulate the approximate time a patient's films may be exposed to the darkroom lighting conditions when opening a full mouth series of film packets aseptically. (See Laboratory Exercise 8, Infection Control and Student Partner Practice.)

1. Obtain one size #2 radiographic film packet.

2. Check posted exposure settings for the dental x-ray machine and set at the lowest possible setting to only slightly expose the silver halide crystals. Slightly exposing the film will prepare the silver halide crystals to react to possible unsafe lighting conditions in the darkroom in the same manner as exposed patient films.

3. Prepare to expose the film by placing it tube side up on the countertop or operatory chair.

4. Direct the PID over the film packet. The goal is to only slightly expose the film, so maintain a distance of 12 inches between the edge of the PID and the film packet.

5. Expose the film at this low exposure setting and 12-inch distance.

6. In the darkroom, secure the door, turn off the overhead white light, and turn on the safelight.

7. Open the pre-exposed film packet and place the film on a paper towel on the counter where patient films will be handled.

8. Place a coin on top of the film. (Figure 13–4 ■)

9. Wait approximately 2 minutes.

10. Remove the coin from the film.

11. Process the film in the usual manner.

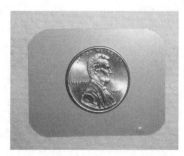

Figure 13–4 Coin test for determining adequacy of the safelight conditions in the darkroom.

Part 3: Quality Control Test for Film Care—Fogged Film Test

The purpose of this activity is to evaluate the condition of film. Whenever a new box of film is opened, it should be tested prior to use. To illustrate what film fogging looks like, use a sample pre-fogged film from your instructor. If a sample of fogged film is not available, you may create a fogged film to use for this exercise.

1. Obtain two size #2 radiographic film packets.
2. Check posted exposure factors for the dental x-ray machine and set at the lowest possible setting.
3. Prepare to slightly expose the film to stray radiation (creating film fog) by placing one of the film packets tube side up on the countertop or operatory chair.
4. Direct the PID over the film packet. Maintain a distance of approximately 12 inches between the edge of the PID and the film packet. Remember that you are only slightly exposing this film.
5. Expose the film at this low exposure setting and 12-inch distance.
6. Do not expose the second film. Do not allow the second film to come in contact with stray radiation, heat, humidity, or chemical fumes.
7. In the darkroom, secure the door, turn off the overhead white light, and turn on the safelight.
8. Process both films.

Part 4: Quality Control Test for Dental X-ray Equipment—Beam Alignment Test

The purpose of this activity is to determine the size and alignment of the primary beam. Use three different metal items to label the films during exposure. Use the Beam Alignment Template that follows to align films for exposure and again after processing to aid in reorienting the exposed radiographs.

1. Obtain four size #2 radiographic film packets.
2. Check posted exposure settings for the dental x-ray machine and set for the maxillary central incisor periapical radiograph.
3. Place the Beam Alignment Template that follows on the countertop or chair designated for this activity. Tear out the Beam Alignment Template from the lab manual and place flat on the countertop.
4. Prepare to expose all four film packets by placing them tube side up on the Beam Alignment Template on the countertop or operatory chair. Position each of the image receptors precisely centered within each of the rectangles drawn to simulate the film packet. Align the embossed dots on each film packet with those drawn on the template. This arrangement will help you identify the radiographs after processing.
5. Place one each of the metal identification objects on three of the films. Record which object you used on the appropriate line on the Beam

Alignment Template. One of the film packets does not need an object placed on it. The images of these objects and the radiograph with no object will further help you identify where to reposition the radiographs back on the template after processing.

6. Direct the PID exactly perpendicular over the center of the Beam Alignment Template. Use the template as your guide to PID placement. Approximately one-half of each of the four films will be in the path of the primary beam. Maintain a distance of 1 inch between the edge of the PID and the film packets placed on the Beam Alignment Template. (Figure 13–5 ■)

7. Expose the films.

8. Process the four films as usual.

9. Using the Beam Alignment Template as a guide, mount each of the four processed radiographs exactly centered within the simulated film mounts regardless of where the exposure circle lines up. (The purpose of this test is to determine if the x-ray beam produced by the x-ray machine is accurate. The circle of radiation exposure that results from your test may NOT align with the circle illustrated on the template.) Use the images of the metal objects to determine the placement of each of the four radiographs.

10. Using a ruler, measure the diameter of the exposure circle created by the four radiographs. Do NOT measure the circle drawn on the template. Measure the diameter of the exposure that resulted from your experiment. Measure across the image and from top to bottom. Record the measurement on the line provided on the template.

Part 5: Quality Control Test for Exposure Consistency— Unit Output Test

The purpose of this activity is to evaluate the dental x-ray machine for consistency of radiation output.

1. Obtain three size #2 radiographic film packets.

2. Check posted exposure settings for the dental x-ray machine and set for the maxillary central incisor periapical radiograph.

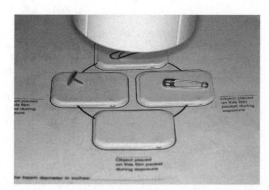

Figure 13–5 Four size #2 film packet image receptors placed on the Beam Alignment Template to determine accuracy of the x-ray beam alignment. Note the arrangement of the metal objects that will help identify the radiographs after processing.

3. Prepare to expose the first film by placing it tube side up on the countertop or operatory chair.

4. Place a step-wedge on top of the film packet.

5. Direct the PID over the film packet and step-wedge. Maintain a distance of 1 inch between the edge of the PID and the film packet-step wedge (Figure 13–3).

6. Expose the first film and step-wedge.

7. Set this exposed film aside.

8. Wait approximately 10 minutes.

9. Expose the second film in the same manner, using the same x-ray machine, at the same settings.

10. Set this second exposed film aside.

11. Wait an additional 10 minutes.

12. Expose the third film in the same manner, using the same x-ray machine, at the same settings.

13. Immediately process all three of the exposed films.

Part 6: Quality Control Test for Digital Image Receptors—Photostimuable Phosphor (PSP) Plate

The purpose of this activity is to evaluate handling of PSP plates after exposure. Following exposure, PSP plates must be protected from bright light until processed in a laser scanner. The manufacturer will usually recommend that the PSP plate be placed into a containment box or on the countertop face down following exposure while awaiting the laser scanning step. Careless exposure of the plates to bright ambient room lighting will compromise the diagnostic quality of the radiographic image.

1. Obtain two size #2 PSP plates.

2. Check posted exposure settings for the dental x-ray machine and set for the maxillary central incisor periapical radiograph.

3. Prepare to expose the PSP plate by placing it tube side up on the countertop or operatory chair.

4. Place a step-wedge on top of the PSP plate.

5. Direct the PID over the PSP plate and step-wedge. Maintain a distance of 1 inch between the edge of the PID and the PSP plate and step-wedge.

6. Expose the first PSP plate and step-wedge.

7. Set this exposed PSP plate aside on the countertop, face up allowing exposure to the overhead room lighting.

8. Wait approximately 10 minutes.

9. Expose the second PSP plate in the same manner, using the same x-ray machine, at the same settings.

10. Take precautions to protect this second PSP plate from overhead room lighting by immediately placing it in the manufacturer's containment box or by immediately placing into the laser scanner.

11. Retrieve the PSP plate exposed first and place into the laser scanner.

12. Observe both images on the computer monitor.

COMPETENCY AND EVALUATION

1. Mount the processed radiographs on the simulated film mounts that follow. Secure with a piece of tape placed along the top edge of the radiograph only, so that the radiographs may be raised slightly to allow light underneath for ease of viewing.

   NOTE: Use the labial mounting method. The raised portion of the embossed dot is toward you (convex) when placing the film onto the page. Observe the digital images obtained using the photostimuable phosphor (PSP) technology on the computer monitor or print out a copy of the images at the direction of your instructor.

2. Place the page with the mounted radiographs taped to it on a viewbox and evaluate. Examine the results of the quality control tests performed in each of the six parts of this exercise. Based on your results, summarize the following in your own words:

   a. Referring to the quality control test performed in Part 1 of this exercise, what is your assessment of the processing chemistry? Why?

   b. Referring to the quality control test performed in Part 2 of this exercise, what is your assessment of the darkroom safelighting? Why?

   c. Referring to the quality control test performed in Part 3 of this exercise, how can you tell that a film is fogged? What effect will film fogging have on the quality of the radiograph?

   d. Referring to the quality control test performed in Part 4 of this exercise, what is your assessment of the x-ray beam of the dental x-ray machine you tested? Why?

   e. Referring to the quality control test performed in Part 5 of this exercise, what is your assessment of the radiation output of the machine you tested? Why?

   f. Referring to the quality control test performed in Part 6 of this exercise, how can you tell that a PSP plate image receptor has been exposed to bright ambient light? What effect will exposure to bright ambient light have on the quality of the radiographic image?

3. Complete the study questions.

Beam Alignment Template

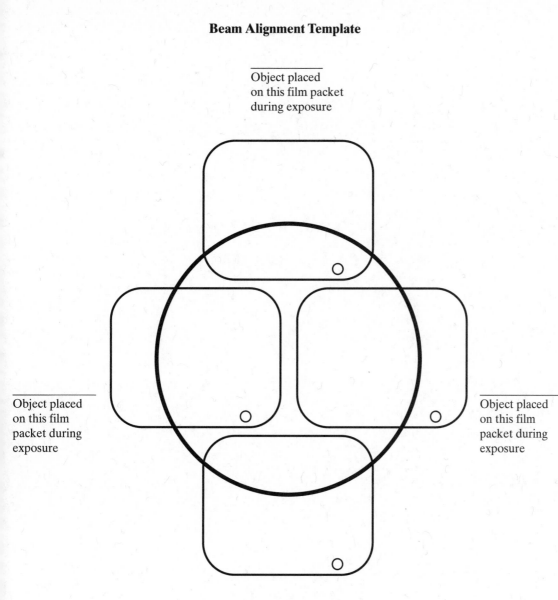

Object placed
on this film packet
during exposure

Object placed
on this film
packet during
exposure

Object placed
on this film
packet during
exposure

Object not required
on this film packet

Record the beam diameter in inches:_____

Part 1

Reference film—processed
at the beginning of the
laboratory session

Film processed at the end
of the laboratory session

Part 2

Coin test to determine
adequacy of the darkroom
safelighting

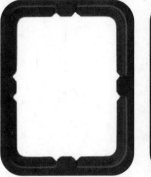
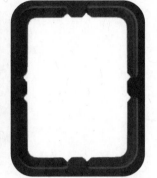
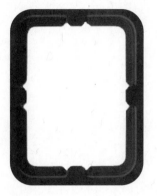

Part 3

Fogged film   Unfogged film

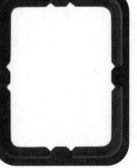

Part 5

Unit output test—mount all 3 films in any order

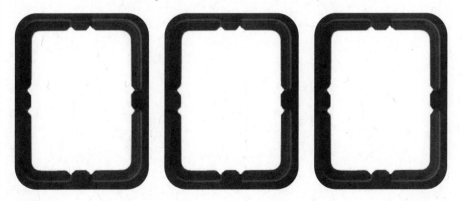

I. Quality assurance
   A. Producing diagnostic quality radiographs while minimizing patient radiation exposure
   B. Quality administration
      1. Responsibility includes the entire oral health care team
         a. Dentist
         b. Dental hygienist
         c. Dental assistant
         d. Qualified expert technician—as required by law
      2. Guidelines for developing and maintaining a quality assurance program
         a. Assess quality assurance needs
         b. Develop quality assurance plan
         c. Assign authority
         d. Provide training
         e. Maintain schedule
         f. Document actions
         g. Evaluate quality assurance plan
   C. Quality control
      1. Specific tests to evaluate quality assurance
         a. Dental x-ray equipment assessment
            1) X-ray unit output test
               a) This test measures the amount of radiation at standard settings over time.
               b) It uses a dosimeter to record output and compare for consistency.
               c) It may also be evaluated using tests with a step-wedge and image receptor.
               d) Image receptors exposed at standard settings over time with a step-wedge can be compared for consistency in density.
               e) A failed test requires attention by qualified expert technician.
            2) X-ray beam collimation test
               a) This test evaluates the beam diameter and alignment.
               b) It uses four size #2 intraoral image receptors, or an extraoral image receptor loaded into a cassette.
               c) Direct the PID over the image receptor(s) and expose.
               d) Evaluate the image for size (beam diameter must be no greater than 2.75 inches (7 cm) and for a distinct edge definition (sharpness).
               e) A failed test requires an inspection of the lead collimator at the base of the PID to ensure that it is seated properly.
            3) Tube head drift assessment (Figure 13–6 ■)
               a) This test evaluates the stability of the tube head in various positions.

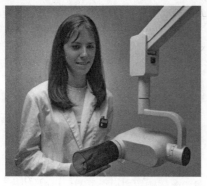

Figure 13–6 Radiographer evaluating the stability of the tube head in various positions.

    b) Extend the support arm and place the tube head in the various positions required to expose all areas of the oral cavity. Observe for drift and/or change of position.

    c) A failed test requires that the support arm be adjusted according to the manufacturer's instructions to eliminate drift and/or vibration.

  b. Dental x-ray film processing equipment

    1) Darkroom adequacy assessment

      a) This test evaluates for white light leak.

      b) It uses a visual inspection.

      c) Enter the darkroom, turn off all lights, including white overhead light and safelighting.

      d) Allow your eyes to become accustomed to the dark, and then visually scan the room for white light leaks.

      e) Check, for example, around doors, pipes, ventilation ducts, and so on.

      f) Use chalk if necessary to mark area of white light leak for location later when white light is turned on.

      g) Inspect darkroom for any other light sources that are not red (safe) in color, such as luminous indicator dials on equipment, luminous wristwatch faces, and so on.

      h) A failed test requires applying a mask or block to the white light leak (Figure 13–7 ■).

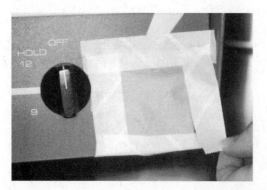

Figure 13–7 Masking a green indicator light on this equipment used in the darkroom to prevent this unsafe lighting from fogging film.

2) Safelight test
   a) This test evaluates the darkroom safelight conditions for the potential to fog film.
   b) It uses the coin test.
   c) Pre-expose an intraoral film to sensitize the silver halide crystals within the emulsion to more realistically simulate films exposed on a patient.
   d) Unwrap the film under safelight conditions.
   e) Place unwrapped film on the darkroom counter and place coin on top of the film to shield this portion of the film from all light in the room (Figure 13–4).
   f) Allow the film to remain on the counter under these conditions for approximately 2 minutes to simulate the amount of time that it would take to aseptically open a full mouth series of films.
   g) Process the film and evaluate for an image of the coin indicating unsafe lighting conditions (Figure 13–8 ■).
   h) A failed test requires an inspection of the condition of the safelight filter, evaluating for scratches, proper seal; also evaluate the filter color (red is appropriate for all dental x-ray film types), bulb wattage (15 watts or less is considered safe for all types of dental x-ray films), distance away from the working area (a minimum of 4 feet above the counter is considered safe for all types of dental x-ray films).
3) Automatic processor function
   a) This test evaluates the adequate setup and function of the automatic processor and processing solutions.
   b) It uses two unexposed intraoral films.
   c) Unwrap one of the unexposed intraoral films under safelight conditions and process normally.
   d) Unwrap one of the unexposed intraoral films under white overhead room lighting (unsafe lighting) and process normally.
   e) When the processing is complete, observe the two films. The film unwrapped under safelight conditions should exit the processor chute dry and clear. The film unwrapped under unsafe white light conditions should exit the processor chute dry and black.

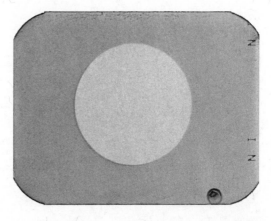

Figure 13–8 Coin test results indicating unsafe light conditions. Note the outline of the coin indicating the area around the coin that was exposed by unsafe light conditions.

    f) A failed test is indicated when these results differ, indicating that the processor be checked for proper setup, such as developer and fixer chemistry in the appropriate tanks and completely full; that the rinse water is turned on; that the dryer is functioning properly. If the cause of failure cannot be determined, a qualified technician should service the machine.

   4) Processing chemistry test

    a) This test evaluates the efficacy of processing chemistry.

    b) It uses a reference film.

    c) Expose several intraoral films (the number of films exposed depends on the usage load on the processing chemistry—30 exposed films may be needed for those practices whose chemistry will probably require changing in 30 days; seven films may be adequate for those practices in which chemistry is changed weekly). Use a step-wedge and expose all of the films with the same x-ray machine at the same settings, one immediately after the other.

    d) Process only one of the exposed films using fresh processing chemistry, store the remaining films in a safe place (away from radiation, heat, humidity, chemical fumes).

    e) Attach the processed radiograph with the step-wedge image to a viewbox. At the beginning of each day, obtain one of the exposed films and process normally; compare each subsequent film to the reference film. The density of each film should match the density observed in the reference film.

    f) A failed test is indicated when the newly processed film image of the step-wedge appears lighter than the reference film, indicating that the processing solutions should be replaced with fresh chemicals.

 c. Dental x-ray film assessment

  1) This is the proper film storage test.

  2) It evaluates the condition of dental x-ray film.

  3) It uses one film from a freshly opened new box.

   a) Open the film under safelight conditions and process normally.

   b) Inspect the processed film for fog.

   c) A failed test requires checking the expiration date on the film box. Use oldest film first to assist in using film prior to expiration date; evaluate the film storage area for possible fogging from radiation, excess heat, and/or humidity, chemical fumes.

 d. Digital image receptor assessment

  1) This evaluates the ability of a solid-state digital sensor or photostimuable phosphor (PSP) plate to record a radiographic image without noise (electronic equivalent of film fog) or missing data (electronic equivalent of scratched or damaged emulsion).

2) It uses visual inspection to assess the image receptor surface for damage, bending, scratches, and for a loose or crimped computer cable/wire.

3) A failed inspection requires replacing the sensor or computer cable/wire.

e. Dental radiograph viewing conditions assessment

   1) Viewbox inspection

      a) This evaluates the condition of the viewbox to enhance interpretation and diagnosis.

      b) It uses visual inspection to assess the viewbox for fluorescent bulb flicker or a color change to black indicating bulb failure.

      c) Visually inspect the viewbox surface for scratches and debris.

      d) A failed inspection requires replacing the bulb and/or cleaning the viewbox surface.

   2) Computer monitor inspection

      a) This inspection evaluates the position of the computer monitor to enhance viewing digital radiographic images.

      b) With the computer monitor in the off position, observe monitor surface for glare from harsh overhead lighting or natural light coming through nearby windows.

      c) A failed test requires repositioning the computer monitor to eliminate or minimize glare.

f. Extraoral dental radiographic assessment

   1) Film cassette inspection

      a) Assess the condition of the cassette to ensure that light cannot leak into the cassette and to ensure a tight contact between film and intensifying screens.

      b) Use a visual inspection to examine the lock/snap mechanism for securing the cassette (Figure 13–9 ■).

      c) A failed assessment requires repairing or replacing the damaged cassette.

   2) Intensifying screens inspection

      a) Evaluate the condition of the intensifying screens to avoid the presence of artifacts, which hinder interpretation and diagnosis.

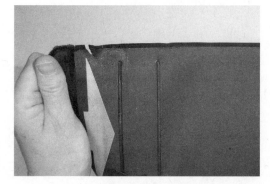

Figure 13–9 Visual inspection of this cassette reveals tears that may be allowing white light to enter the cassette and expose the film.

b) Use a visual inspection of intensifying screens. Look for scratches, debris, or worn areas.

c) A failed test requires cleaning or replacement of the intensifying screens. Avoid overcleaning intensifying screens. Clean only as needed.

II. Documentation

   A. Post instructions

      1. Dental x-ray machine recommended settings should be posted near the control panel to prevent exposure errors.

      2. Processing instructions should be posted in the darkroom to prevent processing errors.

      3. Other procedures such as extraoral radiographic exposures, film duplicating, and film identification methods should have posted instructions.

   B. Maintenance schedule log

      1. Record when each quality control test is due and performed and document the results and corrective action taken (if it was necessary).

      2. Assign maintenance duties and authority.

   C. Maintain an error log

      1. Identify retake errors and corrective action taken and record in writing.

      2. Use this log as a basis for identifying areas that need preventive quality control action.

      3. Use this log as a basis for in-service and retraining personnel.

REFERENCES

Carestream Health Inc. (2007). *Exposure and processing for dental film radiography.* N-413 CAT No. 832 8783. Rochester, NY: Author.

Thomson, E. M., & Johnson, O. N. (2012). *Essentials of dental radiography for dental assistants and hygienists* (9th ed.). Upper Saddle River, NJ: Pearson.

1. The goal of quality assurance is to achieve maximum diagnostic yield from each radiograph.
   Quality control means using tests to ensure quality.
   - A. The first statement is true. The second statement is false.
   - B. The first statement is false. The second statement is true.
   - C. Both statements are true.
   - D. Both statements are false.

2. Who is responsible for administration of a quality assurance program?
   - A. Dentist
   - B. Dental hygienist
   - C. Dental assistant
   - D. All of the above

3. Each of the following is a quality control test for monitoring the dental x-ray machine EXCEPT one. Which one is the EXCEPTION?
   - A. Coin test
   - B. Tube head stability test
   - C. Output consistency test
   - D. Beam alignment test

4. A step-wedge can be used to test each of the following EXCEPT one. Which one is the EXCEPTION?
   - A. X-ray machine output/consistency
   - B. Adequacy of the safelight
   - C. Protection of PSP sensor from light
   - D. Processing chemistry strength

5. Which of the following intraoral dental x-ray machine beam diameters is within acceptable limits?
   - A. 2.75 inches
   - B. 3.75 inches
   - C. 4.75 inches
   - D. 5.75 inches

6. The coin test may be used to determine which of the following?
   - A. Film density
   - B. Processing errors
   - C. Safelight adequacy
   - D. X-ray machine output

7. The outline of the coin recorded on the radiograph as a result of the coin test would indicate?
   - A. A successful test
   - B. A failed test

8. When the automatic processor is functioning properly, an unexposed film opened appropriately under safelight conditions will exit the return chute dry and
   - A. black.
   - B. clear.
   - C. green.
   - D. with the image of a coin.

9. A film processed under ideal conditions and used to compare subsequent radiographic images is called a
   A. fresh film.
   B. fogged film.
   C. duplicate film.
   D. reference film.

10. Each of the following plays a role in quality control of extraoral radiographic cassettes and intensifying screens EXCEPT one. Which one is the EXCEPTION?
    A. Clean with appropriate cleanser after every use.
    B. Check to remove debris periodically.
    C. Perform a visual inspection for scratches.
    D. Replace or repair cassette tears.

laboratory exercise 14

Radiographic Interpretation

INTRODUCTION

Dental hygienists and dental assistants play an important role in interpretation of radiographs. Although it is the dentist's responsibility for the final diagnosis and treatment recommendations, all members of the oral health care team should be able to recognize radiographic deviations from the normal. Patient care is enhanced when radiographs are interpreted, and findings that deviate from normal radiographic anatomy are called to the attention of the dentist. Additionally, the ability to read and explain radiographic findings to the patient is an important skill.

Furthermore, developing interpretation skills fosters an appreciation for obtaining quality radiographs. Knowing what information is being sought from a radiographic image motivates the radiographer to obtain precise images. For example, a slight placement error may at first seem insignificant until compared with accurate placement that reveals disease that would have been misdiagnosed from the incorrectly placed radiograph (Figure 14–1 ■).

Interpretation is a skill that requires practice. The beginner may easily become frustrated by a seeming inability to see what the expert easily identifies. Furthermore, because radiographs are two-dimensional representations of three-dimensional structures, image variations of normal anatomical landmarks can be confusing. Varying radiographic density may also alter the appearance of normal anatomy. For these reasons, it is important to understand that the basis for developing interpretative skills is a solid working knowledge of normal radiographic anatomy. When interpreting a radiographic image, first identify normal anatomy, then systematically

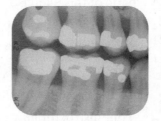 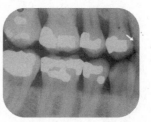

Figure 14–1 The premolar bitewing radiograph on the left was not positioned to image the distal portion of the maxillary canine. When correctly positioned to record the distal portion of the canine, as in the radiograph on the right, caries is now apparent.

progress through an evaluation sequence, assigning a name to every radiopacity and radiolucency observed.

For the purpose of organizing the learning process, this exercise divides the interpretative practice into five categories: (1) tooth development and anomalies, (2) dental materials, (3) periodontal disease, (4) caries, and (5) other common oral conditions. Using a form that guides the interpretative process, you are less likely to omit or not see something that should be identified. It is important to note that successful interpretation begins with a working knowledge of normal anatomy of the maxillofacial region (the dental arches and the supporting facial structures of the head and neck) and various types of dental materials. The purpose of this exercise is to provide systematic practice at learning how to interpret dental radiographs.

OBJECTIVES

Following completion of this lab activity, you will be able to:

1. Identify tooth development and common anomalies radiographically.

2. Identify common dental materials radiographically.

3. Identify evidence of periodontal disease radiographically.

4. Identify deviations in tooth structure that represent suspected caries radiographically.

MATERIALS

Magnifying device

Periodontal probe

Sample patient radiographs

Viewbox (film-based)

Computer monitor (digital images)

PREPARATION

1. Study the chapter outline to prepare for this laboratory exercise. An understanding of the material presented in the outline is required to complete this activity.

2. View the images of the radiographs that accompany each of the four parts of this exercise.

3. Using the Radiographic Interpretation Form appropriate for each of the four parts, document your interpretation of the radiographs. Note that not all conditions are present on the sample radiographs provided. Nevertheless, it is important that radiographs be examined for the presence of all possible conditions.

4. Your instructor may provide you with additional sample radiographs. The Radiographic Interpretation Forms may be copied and used to

interpret the patient radiographs for additional practice, or you may be directed to use the interpretation form available at your facility.

    a. Designate an area with a viewbox (film-based) or computer monitor (digital).
    b. Dim overhead bright room lighting.
    c. Use a magnifying glass, periodontal probe (film-based), or the software magnification and measurement tools (digital).
    d. Limit beginning interpretation sessions to 30 minutes to avoid eye fatigue.

LABORATORY EXERCISE ACTIVITIES

Part 1: Interpretation—Tooth Development and Abnormalities

View the radiographs, and, using the Radiographic Interpretation Form—Tooth Development and Abnormalities, record findings.

Part 2: Interpretation—Dental Materials

View the radiographs, and, using the Radiographic Interpretation Form—Dental Materials, record findings.

Part 3: Interpretation—Periodontal Disease

View the radiographs, and, using the Radiographic Interpretation Form—Periodontal Disease, record findings.

Part 4: Interpretation—Caries

View the radiographs, and, using the Radiographic Interpretation Form—Caries, record findings.

Part 5: Interpretation—Sample Radiographs

View the radiographs provided by your instructor, and, using the Radiographic Interpretation Forms from Parts 1 to 4 or a form supplied by your instructor, record findings.

COMPETENCY AND EVALUATION

1. Did using a form help you proceed through the interpretive process? In what ways did the simulated forms presented here, or the form your instructor gave you, guide you through the interpretive process?

2. Compare your completed forms with other students in the class. Did you identify the same conditions or do your interpretations differ? In what ways?

3. Complete the study questions.

Part 1: Tooth Development and Anomalies

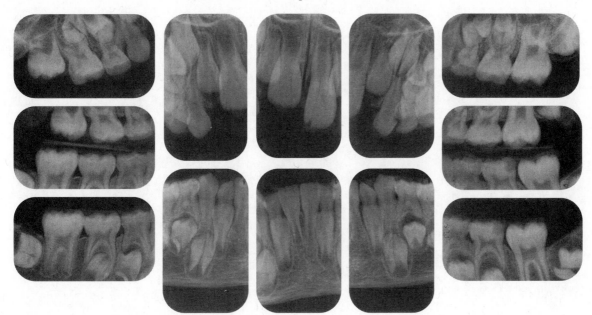

Radiographic Interpretation Form—Tooth Development and Anomalies

View the radiographs for evidence of the conditions listed in the column at the right. Begin the interpretation process in the maxillary right. View tooth #1 (maxillary right third molar) and vicinity. If tooth #1 is not present radiographically, "X" out the tooth number and begin the interpretation process with tooth #2 (maxillary right second molar). If tooth #1 is present radiographically, circle the tooth number and then proceed to evaluate tooth #1 for the conditions listed in the column on the right. Evaluate both permanent and primary teeth and vicinity for these conditions.

Condition present:

Tooth # 1 2 3 4 5 6 7 8 9 10 11 12 13 14 15 16 17 18 19 20 21 22 23 24 25 26 27 28 29 30 31 32

- Unerupted/impacted
- Congenitally missing/supernumerary
- Fusion/gemination
- Taurodontia/pulp stones
- Root dilaceration/supernumerary root
- Dens en dente/enamel pearl
- Macrodontia/microdontia
- External resorption/internal resorption

Tooth # A B C D E F G H I J K L M N O P Q R S T

- Unerupted/impacted
- Congenitally missing/supernumerary
- Fusion/gemination
- Taurodontia/pulp stones
- Root dilaceration/supernumerary root
- Dens en dente/enamel pearl
- Macrodontia/microdontia
- External resorption/internal resorption
- Other

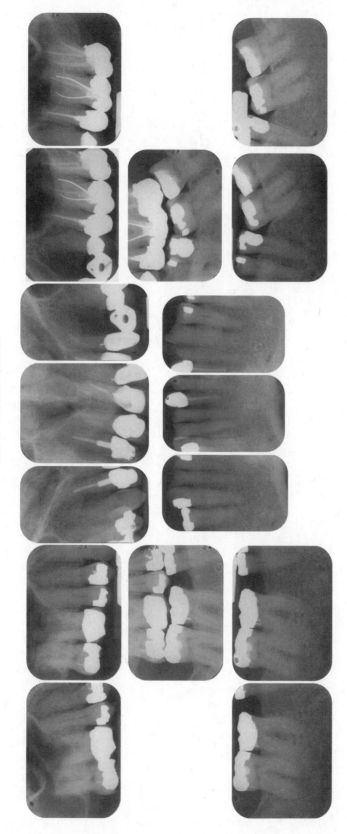

Part 2: Dental Materials

Radiographic Interpretation Form — Dental Materials

View the radiographs for the presence of these restorative materials. Begin the interpretation process in the maxillary right. View tooth #1 (maxillary right third molar). If tooth #1 is not present radiographically, "X" out the tooth number and begin the interpretation process with tooth #2 (maxillary right second molar). If tooth #1 is present radiographically, circle the tooth number and then proceed to evaluate tooth #1 for the presence of any of the materials listed in the column on the right. Check all materials present. (For example, tooth #1 may have a metallic crown, endodontic filling, and also be an abutment.)

Dental materials present:

Tooth #	1	2	3	4	5	6	7	8	9	10	11	12	13	14	15	16	17	18	19	20	21	22	23	24	25	26	27	28	29	30	31	32	
Metallic restoration (amalgam)																																	
Metallic crown (gold, semi-precious metal)																																	
Stainless steel crown																																	
Porcelain fused to metal crown																																	
Porcelain crown (porcelain jacket, veneer)																																	
Composite restoration (silicate, acrylic)																																	
Temporary restoration																																	
Sealant																																	
Base material																																	
Cement																																	
Retention pin																																	
Post and core																																	
Endodontic filling (gutta percha, silver points)																																	
Implant																																	
Orthodontic appliance																																	
Abutment																																	
Pontic																																	
Other (foreign object such as amalgam tatoo, facial jewelry, etc.)																																	

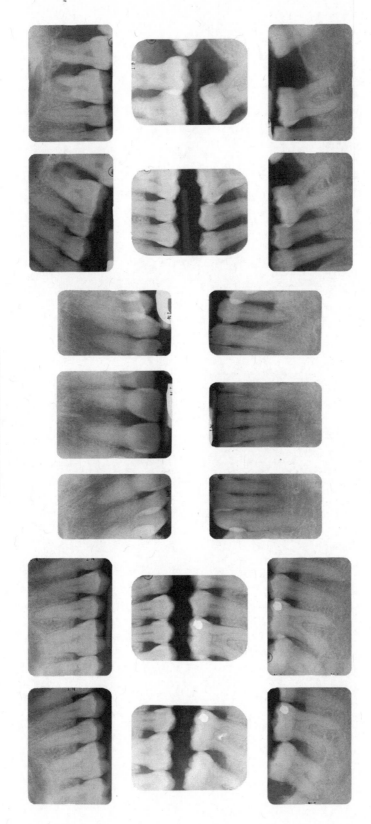

Part 3: Periodontal Disease

Radiographic Interpretation Form — Periodontal Disease

View the radiographs for evidence of periodontal disease and local contributing factors. Begin the interpretation process in the maxillary right. View tooth #1 (maxillary right third molar). If tooth #1 is not present radiographically out the tooth number and begin the interpretation process with tooth #2 (maxillary right second molar). If tooth #1 is present radiographically, circle the tooth number and then proceed to evaluate tooth #1 for evidence of any of the conditions listed in the column on the right. Check all conditions present. (For example, tooth #1 may have calculus present, bone loss, and furcation involvement.)

Tooth #

Periodontal condition present:

Tooth #	Calculus	Overhanging or defective restoration or poorly contoured crown margins	Open contact	Widening of PDL space	Triangulation	Early bone loss (indistinct lamina dura, fuzzy radiolucency in crestal bone area)	Moderate bone loss (distinct cupping out of the crestal bone, 30–50% loss compared to length of tooth root)	Advanced bone loss (crestal bone loss is >50% compared to length of tooth root)	Horizontal bone loss	Vertical bone loss	Furcation involvement	Evidence of tooth mobility (drift)	Periodontal abscess	Other (specify)
1														
2														
3														
4														
5														
6														
7														
8														
9														
10														
11														
12														
13														
14														
15														
16														
17														
18														
19														
20														
21														
22														
23														
24														
25														
26														
27														
28														
29														
30														
31														
32														

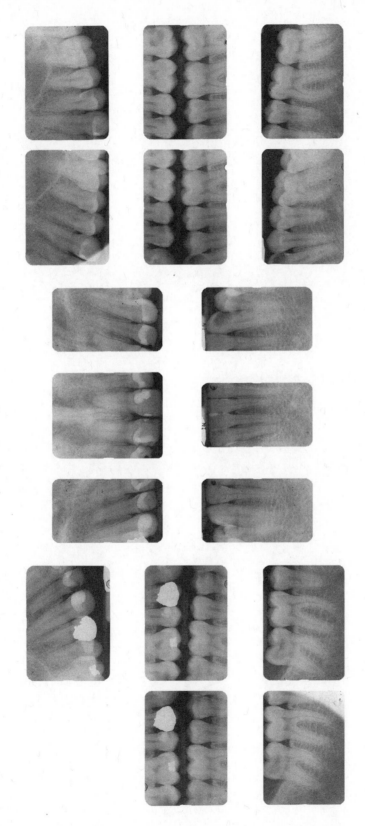

Part 4: Caries

Radiographic Interpretation Form — Caries

View the radiographs for evidence of caries and defective restorations. Begin the interpretation process in the maxillary right. View tooth #1 (maxillary right third molar). If tooth #1 is not present radiographically, "X" out the tooth number and begin the interpretation process with tooth #2 (maxillary right second molar). If tooth #1 is present radiographically, circle the tooth number and then proceed to evaluate tooth #1 for evidence of any of the conditions listed in the column on the right. Remember that cervical burnout, abrasion, attrition, and erosion may all mimic decay. Do not record these conditions, and do not confuse them with caries.

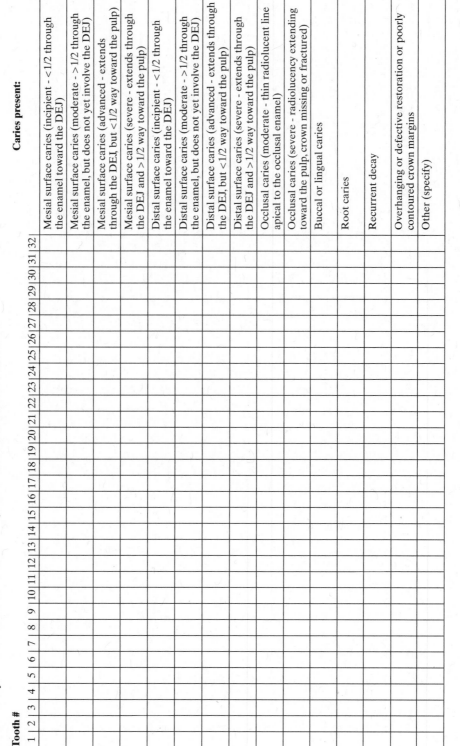

Tooth #

Caries present:

Tooth #	1	2	3	4	5	6	7	8	9	10	11	12	13	14	15	16	17	18	19	20	21	22	23	24	25	26	27	28	29	30	31	32
Mesial surface caries (incipient - <1/2 through the enamel toward the DEJ)																																
Mesial surface caries (moderate - >1/2 through the enamel, but does not yet involve the DEJ)																																
Mesial surface caries (advanced - extends through the DEJ, but <1/2 way toward the pulp)																																
Mesial surface caries (severe - extends through the DEJ and >1/2 way toward the pulp)																																
Distal surface caries (incipient - <1/2 through the enamel toward the DEJ)																																
Distal surface caries (moderate - >1/2 through the enamel, but does not yet involve the DEJ)																																
Distal surface caries (advanced - extends through the DEJ, but <1/2 way toward the pulp)																																
Distal surface caries (severe - extends through the DEJ and >1/2 way toward the pulp)																																
Occlusal caries (moderate - thin radiolucent line apical to the occlusal enamel)																																
Occlusal caries (severe - radiolucency extending toward the pulp, crown missing or fractured)																																
Buccal or lingual caries																																
Root caries																																
Recurrent decay																																
Overhanging or defective restoration or poorly contoured crown margins																																
Other (specify)																																

I. Radiographic interpretation
- A. Interpretation skills are required by the
  1. Dental assistant
  2. Dental hygienist
  3. Dentist
- B. Requirements
  1. Thorough knowledge of normal radiographic anatomy
  2. Quality radiographs
  3. Mounted anatomically correct
     - a. This provides systematic viewing.
     - b. Opaque film mounts block extraneous light to aid viewing.
  4. Light source
     - a. Subdued overhead room lighting
     - b. Viewbox (film-based radiographs)
     - c. Computer monitor placement to avoid glare (digital images)
  5. Magnification
  6. Probe (film-based radiographs) or software measuring tool (digital imaging)
- C. Systematic viewing
  1. Examine the entire radiograph.
  2. Begin the examination on the maxillary right side, proceed to the maxillary left, then to the mandibular left, and finish examination on the mandibular right.
  3. Use adjacent radiographs to compare views.
  4. Use a chart or diagram to record each of the following:
     - a. Presence or absence of teeth
     - b. Anomalies such as impactions, unerupted or transposed teeth, congenitally missing teeth
     - c. Dental materials (if present)
     - d. Evidence of periodontal disease
       1) Note alveolar bone height.
       2) Identify local contributing factors such as calculus and overhanging restorations.
       3) Examine the periodontal ligament space, document abnormal widening, triangulation.
     - e. Deviations in tooth structure that represent suspected caries
       1) View all surfaces of each tooth.
       2) Examine the contact point for proximal decay.
       3) Examine restoration margins for recurrent decay.
       4) Examine the area just apical to the enamel for occlusal decay.
       5) Examine for buccal/lingual decay.
       6) Examine for root decay if conditions such as bone loss or tooth extrusion exist.
     - f. Oral pathology
       1) Identify and examine every anatomic structure; assign a name to each radiopacity and radiolucency; note when some part of the image cannot be identified.

    2) Examine the bone around each tooth, noting density and trabecular pattern; compare with views in adjacent radiographs and compare left and right sides for symmetry.

    3) Examine the periodontal ligament space, observing asymmetry or breaks in the continuity.

    4) Examine the pulp chamber of each tooth; look for changes in density.

5. Record substantive radiographic deviations from the norm, documenting location, size, shape, borders, symmetry, and density.

6. Use a probe (film-based radiographs) or software measuring tool (digital images).

7. Use radiographs exposed previously for comparison.

  a. Compare to previous radiographs only after a thorough evaluation of the current radiographs.

  b. Do not allow previous radiographs to influence or prejudice the initial interpretation of the current radiographs.

II. Radiographic appearance of tooth development and anomalies

A. Advantages of the use of radiographs in evaluating tooth development and detecting anomalies

1. Assessment of growth and development

2. Detection of asymptomatic abnormalities

3. Documentation of the patient's condition at a specific point in time

B. Considerations when using radiographs in evaluating tooth development and detecting anomalies

1. Radiographic findings should be utilized in conjunction with the clinical examination.

2. Two-dimensional radiographs of three-dimensional structures may miss or mimic a developmental anomaly.

C. Tooth development

1. Dental sac appears as a circular radiolucency

2. Enamel cusps are the first to calcify and appear radiopaque.

3. The crown develops as a radiopacity surrounded by a radiolucent follicle.

4. The crown erupts as roots continue to form.

5. Roots first appear open, dental papilla.

  a. Dental papilla should not be confused with periapical pathology.

  b. Differentiate from a periapical lesion by the age of the patient and stage of tooth development and by the presence of a contributing condition such as a large carious lesion.

6. Root apices close, completing tooth development.

D. Tooth eruption patterns

1. Various stages of tooth development may be visible.

2. Permanent tooth development causes resorption of the primary tooth roots.

3. First, second, third permanent molars do not have primary predecessors.

4. Supernumerary teeth may be detected.

5. Congenitally missing teeth may be detected.

6. Variations in tooth roots may be detected, such as:
   a. Supernumerary roots
   b. Dilacerated roots
7. Malpositioned/transposed teeth can be observed.

E. Anomalies
   1. Macrodontia
      a. Appears as a larger-than-normal tooth
      b. Differentiate from image magnification
   2. Microdontia
      a. Appears as a smaller-than-normal tooth
      b. More common occurrence in maxillary lateral incisors (peg laterals) and the third molars
   3. Gemination
      a. Appears as two crowns fused together sharing one root and root canal structure
      b. Differentiate from fusion by identifying the presence of the adjacent teeth
   4. Fusion
      a. Appears as two crowns and two root and root canal structures fused together
      b. Differentiate from gemination by identifying the absence of an adjacent tooth
   5. Concrescence
      a. Teeth appear joined by cementum
      b. Very difficult to diagnose radiographically
      c. Teeth with roots in close proximity and/or the angle of the x-ray beam often mimic this anomaly.
   6. Dens invaginatus
      a. Appearance of a "tooth within a tooth"
      b. Invagination of enamel within the pulp chamber
   7. Enamel pearl
      a. Appears as a radiopaque sphere attached to the tooth surface in the cervical region
      b. Differentiate from pulp stone by its location outside of the pulp chamber
   8. Taurodontism
      a. Appears as an enlarged pulp chamber, resembling a bull (tauros–bull; odont–tooth)
      b. Usually affects mandibular molar teeth

III. Radiographic appearance of dental materials
   A. Advantages of the use of radiographs in identifying and evaluating dental materials
      1. Document the condition of restoration margins.
      2. Assess past dental procedures such as endodontic therapy, apicoectomy, and extraction sites.
      3. Aid in documentation, dental charting.
   B. Considerations when using radiographs to identify and evaluate dental materials
      1. Some dental materials are not readily distinguishable radiographically.
      2. Some dental materials may mimic caries.

C. Radiopaque
   1. Amalgam
      a. This can be differentiated from other materials by irregular margins.
      b. It may cover one or multiple surfaces of the tooth crown.
      c. Amalgam tattoo may appear as a radiopaque metal scrap outside the tooth, embedded in soft tissue.
   2. Metal crown
      a. This can be differentiated from other materials by smooth margins.
      b. It usually covers entire tooth crown.
      c. Gold cannot be distinguished radiographically from other semiprecious metals.
      d. A stainless steel crown may appear less radiopaque with a "see-through" appearance.
      e. Porcelain, which appears less radiopaque than metal, may be visible in a porcelain fused-to-metal crown.
   3. Gold onlay and inlay
      a. Difficult to distinguish from other metal restorations
      b. Usually appears to have smooth, regular margins
      c. Does not usually cover the entire tooth crown
   4. Composite
      a. Less radiopaque than metal restorations
      b. Radiopacity similar to dentin
   5. Porcelain
      a. This is less radiopaque than metal restorations.
      b. Its radiopacity is similar to dentin.
      c. It may be used in porcelain fused-to-metal crowns, where the porcelain may be visible on the incisal/occlusal edge beyond the metal portion of the crown.
      d. When used as a single material, prepared tooth is visible beneath the porcelain crown.
   6. Temporary filling material
      a. This is less radiopaque than metal restorations.
      b. Its radiopacity is similar to dentin.
      c. Irregular margins help differentiate this from composite.
   7. Base material
      a. Radiopacity similar to dentin
      b. May require close examination under the margin of large amalgam or composite restoration to detect radiographically
   8. Cement
      a. Radiopacity varies, may appear as radiopaque as a metal
      b. When visible radiographically, usually appears beneath a porcelain crown
   9. Sealant
      a. Radiopacity very similar to dentin; not usually detected radiographically
      b. Requires careful examination of the area just beneath the occlusal enamel to detect radiographically
  10. Retention pin
      a. Differentiate from other materials by shape

      b. Unique shape easily distinguishable.

      c. May require a close examination near margin of large restorations to detect

      d. Appears embedded in the enamel only; will not perforate the pulp chamber

11. Post and core

      a. This can be differentiated from other materials by shape.

      b. Its unique shape is usually easily distinguishable.

      c. Location in pulp chamber helps distinguish this material from retention pin.

      d. If post and core present, tooth must also have had endodontic therapy.

12. Silver points

      a. Differentiate from other materials by shape and location

      b. Located in root canals

      c. More radiopaque than gutta percha

13. Gutta percha

      a. Differentiate from other materials by shape and location

      b. Located in root canals

      c. Less radiopaque than silver points

14. Implant

      a. Differentiate from other materials by shape and location

      b. Located in area of missing tooth/teeth

      c. Appears imbedded in alveolar bone

      d. Restoration; usually crown and/or crown and bridge attached

15. Fixed orthodontic appliances

      a. Differentiate from other materials by shape and location

      b. Unique shape usually easily distinguishable

D. Radiolucent

  1. Composites, silicate, acrylic

      a. Older restorative materials may appear radiolucent.

      b. Regular margins that appear prepared and location in the anterior teeth help differentiate composite from caries.

  2. Radiopaque fillers are added to modern-day dental materials that would be likely to appear radiolucent or less radiopaque so that these can be readily distinguished radiographically.

IV. Radiographic appearance of evidence of periodontal disease

A. Advantages of the use of radiographs in the evaluation of periodontal health

  1. Images the condition of supporting bone

  2. Locates the presence of local contributing factors such as calculus and overhanging restorations

  3. Aids in treatment planning and implementation by identifying infrabony defects, tooth morphology

  4. Aids in prognosis by imaging root-to-crown ratio

B. Considerations when using radiographs in the evaluation of periodontal health

  1. Radiographs do not image early changes in the periodontium.

  2. Actual destruction of periodontal tissue is more advanced than can be recorded radiographically.

  3. Two-dimensional image may hide infrabony defects.

4. Soft-to-hard tissue ratio not imaged.
5. One cannot distinguish between active and inactive disease status.
- C. Radiographic techniques
  1. Paralleling technique
     a. Parallel central ray of the x-ray beam records alveolar bone more accurately than bisecting technique.
     b. Bitewing radiographs, particularly vertical bitewing radiographs, provide an accurate representation of the alveolar bone.
     c. Periapical radiographs require precise vertical angulation to achieve the accurate representation of the alveolar bone recorded with bitewing radiographs.
  2. A higher kilovoltage (kVp) setting that produces a long scale (low contrast) image is purported to be best at recording subtle changes in the periodontium. In practice evaluating periodontal disease occurs equally well from long scale as short scale (high contrast) images.
- D. Local contributing factors that can be recorded on radiographs
  1. Calculus
  2. Overhanging restorations
  3. Occlusal trauma evidenced by widening of the periodontal ligament space
- E. Radiographic appearance of health or gingivitis (American Academy of Periodontology Case Type I)
  1. Interproximal alveolar bone appears within 1.5 to 2 mm below the cemento-enamel junction.
  2. Lamina dura visible and radiopaque.
  3. Crestal bone pointed in the anterior region; horizontal and intersects the tooth at 90-degree angle in the posterior region.
- F. Radiographic appearance of slight chronic periodontitis (American Academy of Periodontology Case Type II)
  1. There is loss of density in the alveolar crest area.
  2. Interproximal bone in the anterior region appears slightly less pointed; there is indistinct fuzziness in the posterior region.
  3. Triangulation (widening of the periodontal ligament space at the alveolar crest) may be present.
- G. Radiographic appearance of moderate chronic or aggressive periodontitis (American Academy of Periodontology Case Type III)
  1. Alveolar bone loss appears to be 30–50 percent when compared with the tooth root length.
  2. Crestal bone loss may be horizontally or vertically patterned.
  3. Radiolucencies between the roots of multirooted teeth may indicate furcation involvement.
- H. Radiographic appearance of advanced chronic or aggressive periodontitis (American Academy of Periodontology Case Type IV)
  1. This can be easily recognized radiographically.
  2. Alveolar bone loss appears to be greater than 50 percent when compared with the tooth root length.
  3. Furcation involvement is usually evident.
  4. Tooth movement may be evident radiographically as shifted or displaced teeth.

V. Radiographic appearance of deviations in tooth structure that represent suspected caries
   A. Advantages of the use of radiographs in the detection of caries
      1. Images proximal surface caries that cannot be detected clinically
      2. Images the extent of caries
   B. Considerations when using radiographs in the detection of caries
      1. Caries are usually more advanced than the radiograph can record.
      2. Occlusal, buccal, and lingual caries are not imaged until moderately advanced.
      3. Other conditions, such as abrasion, attrition, and radiolucent composite restorative materials may mimic caries.
      4. Optical illusions, such as cervical burnout and mach banding, interfere with caries detection.
         a. Cervical burnout is often observed at the mesial and distal root surfaces at the cemento-enamel junction as a radiolucency caused by the concave shape of the root.
         b. Mach banding is often observed along the borders of sharp contrast, such as around areas of slight overlapping between adjacent teeth.
   C. Radiographic techniques
      1. Paralleling technique
         a. Parallel central ray of the x-ray beam records the proximal surface contact area more accurately than bisecting technique.
         b. Bitewing radiographs provide an accurate representation of the proximal surface contact area.
         c. Periapical radiographs require precise vertical angulation to achieve the accurate representation of the interproximal contact area achieved with bitewing radiographs.
      2. A lower kilovoltage (kVp) setting that produces a short-scale (high contrast) image is purported to be best at recording subtle radiolucent changes in radiopaque enamel. In practice evaluating evidence of suspected caries occurs equally well from short-scale as long-scale (low contrast) images.
   D. Proximal surface caries
      1. This appears at or just apical to the proximal surface contact area.
      2. When bone loss is present or tooth extrusion has occurred, it may appear on the root surface.
      3. Proximal surface caries grading system (suggested by Haugejorden and Slack, 1977)
         a. C-1 Incipient
            1) Appears as a radiolucent notch
            2) Penetrates less than halfway through the enamel
         b. C-2 Moderate
            1) Appears as a radiolucent triangle
            2) Penetrates more than halfway through the enamel but does not reach the dentin-enamel junction
         c. C-3 Advanced
            1) Appears as two radiolucent triangles

<ul>
<li style="list-style:none">
<ul>
<li style="list-style:none">
<ul>
<li style="list-style:none">
2) Penetrates the dentin-enamel junction but does not reach more than halfway to the pulp

d. C-4 Severe
<ul>
<li style="list-style:none">
1) Appears as two radiolucent triangles or a large, diffuse radiolucency
2) Penetrates the dentin-enamel junction and reaches more than halfway to the pulp
</li>
</ul>
</li>
</ul>
</li>
</ul>
</li>
</ul>

E. Buccal/lingual caries
1. Appears as a round radiolucency in the center of the tooth crown
2. Cannot differentiate between buccal and lingual location of carious lesion on a two-dimensional radiograph

F. Occlusal caries
1. Appears as a radiolucency just apical to the occlusal enamel
2. Usually not visible radiographically until moderately advanced

G. Root caries
1. Appears as a notched or triangular-shaped radiolucency on the proximal surface at or below the cemento-enamel junction
2. Bone loss or tooth extrusion usually evident, indicating an exposed root surface

H. Recurrent decay
1. Appears as a radiolucency adjacent to a restoration margin.
2. Indirect pulp capping may mimic recurrent decay.
   a. Indirect pulp capping appears as a radiolucent shadow adjacent to a restoration.
   b. It indicates where a sedative base and permanent restoration were placed over decay that was not excavated to avoid exposing the pulp.

VI. Radiographic appearance of common oral pathologic conditions

A. Advantages of the use of radiographs in the detection of common oral pathologic conditions
1. Detects asymptomatic abnormalities
2. Locates lesions that cannot be detected clinically

B. Considerations when using radiographs in the detection of common oral pathologic conditions
1. Radiographic findings should be utilized in conjunction with the clinical examination.
2. Two-dimensional radiographs of three-dimensional structures may miss or mimic a pathologic condition.

C. Pulpal changes
1. Resorption
   a. Internal resorption
      1) Appears as a radiolucent widening of the pulp chamber
      2) Differentiate from external resorption by the widening of the pulp chamber
   b. External resorption
      1) Appears as shortened or blunted root structure when resorption begins at the apex
      2) May also appear as a round or diffuse radiolucency on the tooth root

          3) Differentiate from internal resorption by the unaffected root canal

    2. Pulp stone

       a. Appears as a radiopaque sphere in the pulp chamber

       b. Differentiate from enamel pearl by its location inside of the pulp chamber

    3. Pulpal sclerosis

       a. Appears as a narrowing or disappearance of the pulp chamber

       b. Appearance of secondary dentin

D. Periapical lesions

    1. Radiolucent

       a. Abscess, cyst, granuloma

          1) Initially appear as a widening of the periodontal ligament space

          2) Develops into a circular radiolucency at the apex of the tooth

          3) Cannot be distinguished from each other from a radiograph alone

       b. Mental foramen (normal anatomy)

          1) May mimic an abscess or cyst especially when imaged at the root tip of the mandibular second or first premolar

          2) Differentiate from apical pathology by the location of the lamina dura and the periodontal ligament space.

             a) The lamina dura and the periodontal ligament space appear in the normal location, closely outlining the tooth root, when the observed radiolucency is the mental foramen.

             b) The lamina dura and the periodontal ligament space appear to extend away from the normal location and do not closely outline the tooth root, but rather seem to outline the observed radiolucency when the most likely interpretation is apical pathology.

    2. Radiopaque

       a. Condensing osteitis

          1) Appears as a diffuse or circular radiopacity near the apices of a nonvital tooth.

          2) Differentiate from sclerotic bone by the history of prolonged inflammation associated with the tooth present

          3) Differentiate from hypercementosis by the presence of the periodontal ligament space; condensing osteitis does not appear to be attached to the tooth

       b. Sclerotic bone

          1) Appears as a diffuse or circular radiopacity not associated with prolonged inflammation of a tooth

          2) Differentiate from condensing osteitis by the absence of chronic inflammation of the tooth present

          3) Differentiate from hypercementosis by the presence of the periodontal ligament space; sclerotic bone does not appear to be attached to the tooth

       c. Hypercementosis

          1) Appears as an overgrowth of cementum.

2) Roots appear enlarged and bulbous.

3) Differentiate between hypercementosis and condensing osteitis by the presence of the lamina dura and periodontal ligament space, which outline and surround the hypercementosis and separate the tooth root from the alveolar bone.

E. Other cysts
 1. Residual cyst
    a. Appears as a round, ovoid radiolucency
    b. Differentiates from other cysts by the location in an extraction site
 2. Dentigerous cyst
    a. Appears as a round, ovoid radiolucency surrounding the crown only of an unerupted tooth
    b. Differentiate from the normal developing tooth and dental sac by the extent and size of the radiolucency

F. Periapical cemental dysplasia
 1. Early lesion appears radiolucent.
 2. Middle stage lesion appears as a mixed radiolucent and radiopaque mass.
 3. Mature lesion appears radiopaque with slight radiolucent "halo" effect.
 4. It is usually located in the mandibular anterior region.

G. Odontoma
 1. Appears as a group of radiopaque toothlike lesions representing various formations of hard dental tissue (enamel, cementum, dentin)
 2. Usually associated with an unerupted tooth

H. Other conditions that may be observed on a radiograph
 1. Trauma
    a. Fracture appears as a radiolucent break in the root or crown of the tooth.
    b. Erosion appears as an increased radiolucency of the tooth crowns.
    c. Attrition appears as an increased radiolucency of the occlusal/incisal surface.
    d. Abrasion, when located near the cervical area, appears as a notched or triangular radiolucency that may mimic caries.
 2. Foreign materials
    a. Materials accidentally lodged in the soft or hard tissue, such as amalgam or orthodontic wires
    b. The presence of facial jewelry, such as tongue and lip piercing
    c. Metal objects appear radiopaque

REFERENCES

Hatrick, C. D., Eakle, W. S., & Bird, W. F. (2010). *Dental materials: Clinical applications for dental assistants and dental hygienists* (2nd ed.). St. Louis, MO: Elsevier.

Langlais, R. P. (2003). *Exercises in oral radiology and interpretation* (4th ed.). Philadelphia: Saunders.

Perry, D. A., Beemsterboer, P., & Taggart, E. J. (2007). *Periodontology for the dental hygienist,* (3rd ed.). St. Louis, MO: Elsevier.

Thomson, E. M., & Johnson, O. N. (2012). *Essentials of dental radiography for dental assistants and hygienists* (9th ed.). Upper Saddle River, NJ: Pearson.

Thomson, E. M., & Tolle, L. (1994). A practical guide for using radiographs in the assessment of periodontal diseases. Part I: Technique. *Pract Hyg, 3,* 11–16.

Thomson, E. M., & Tolle, S. L. (1994). A practical guide for using radiographs in the assessment of periodontal disease, Part 2: Interpretation and Future Advances. *Pract Hyg, 3,* 2.

White, S. C., & Pharoah, M. J. (2008). *Oral radiology principles and interpretation* (6th ed.). St. Louis, MO: Elsevier.

1. Each of the following is a useful aid when interpreting film-based dental radiographs EXCEPT one. Which one is the EXCEPTION?
   - A. Viewbox
   - B. Magnifying glass
   - C. Bright room lighting
   - D. Film mount

2. A maxillary anterior periapical radiograph reveals shorter-than-normal root lengths on the maxillary lateral incisor. Which of the following is the most likely interpretation?
   - A. External resorption
   - B. Microdontia
   - C. Pulpal sclerosis
   - D. Root fracture

3. A 63-year-old patient has no symptoms. A mandibular periapical radiograph reveals ovoid radiopacities located in the pulp chambers of the mandibular molars. Which of the following is the most likely interpretation?
   - A. Cysts
   - B. Hyperdontia
   - C. Pulp stones
   - D. Supernumerary teeth

4. Which of the following dental materials would appear radiolucent radiographically?
   - A. Acrylic
   - B. Amalgam
   - C. Implant
   - D. Metallic crown

5. Which of the following is a limitation of radiographs in evaluating periodontal disease?
   - A. Estimating bone loss
   - B. Locating contributing factors
   - C. Determining prognosis
   - D. Differentiating between active and inactive disease status

6. An early periodontal health change is seen radiographically as
   - A. An enlargement of the gingiva
   - B. Furcation involvement
   - C. Loss of density of alveolar crest
   - D. Vertical bone loss

7. Each of the following may resemble caries radiographically EXCEPT one. Which one is the EXCEPTION?
   - A. Abrasion
   - B. Attrition
   - C. Cervical burnout
   - D. Metallic restoration

8. Interproximal caries frequently appears radiographically on which area of the tooth?
   A. At or just apical to the gingival margin
   B. At or just apical to the proximal contact point
   C. At or just apical to the occlusal/incisal edge
   D. At or just apical to the cemento-enamel junction

9. A periapical abscess and a periapical cyst can be differentiated on a radiograph by
   A. whether lesion margins are diffuse or well demarcated.
   B. the presence or absence of associated tooth root resorption.
   C. the size and shape of the radiolucency.
   D. abscess and cysts cannot be differentiated from the radiograph alone.

10. A radiolucent oval seen near the apex of the mandibular second premolars that may mimic periapical pathology is
    A. cervical burnout.
    B. mental foramen.
    C. mandibular foramen.
    D. lingual foramen.

Answers to Study Questions

LABORATORY EXERCISE 1
Introduction to Radiation Safety and Dental Radiographic Equipment

1. A	5. C	9. C
2. C	6. A	10. B
3. D	7. D	
4. B	8. C	

LABORATORY EXERCISE 2
Bitewing Radiographic Technique

1. C	5. A	9. B
2. C	6. A	10. D
3. D	7. D	
4. B	8. C	

LABORATORY EXERCISE 3
Introduction to Digital Radiography

1. B	5. A	9. C
2. D	6. D	10. E
3. A	7. C	
4. C	8. B	

LABORATORY EXERCISE 4
Periapical Radiographs—Paralleling Technique

1. C	5. B	9. B
2. B	6. A	10. C
3. C	7. A	
4. D	8. B	

LABORATORY EXERCISE 5
Periapical Radiographs—Bisecting Technique

1. B
2. D
3. A
4. A
5. B
6. B
7. B
8. B
9. C

10. Essay—See outline for key points in Exercises 4 and 5 to be included in this answer.

LABORATORY EXERCISE 6
Mounting and Radiographic Landmarks

1. A
2. A
3. B
4. A
5. C
6. B
7. D
8. B
9. A
10. A

LABORATORY EXERCISE 7
Identifying and Correcting Radiographic Errors

1. E
2. C
3. A
4. B
5. A
6. E
7. D
8. D
9. B

10. Essay—Refer to the outline for key points and reflect on your laboratory experience to answer this question.

LABORATORY EXERCISE 8
Infection Control and Student Partner Practice

1. A
2. B
3. C
4. D
5. D
6. B
7. A
8. D
9. C

10. Essay—See outline for key points to be included in this answer.

LABORATORY EXERCISE 9
Patient Management and Student Partner Practice

1. D
2. C
3. A
4. B
5. B
6. C
7. A
8. D
9. A

10. Essay—Reflect on your laboratory experience to evaluate your progress.

LABORATORY EXERCISE 10
Occlusal Radiographic Techniques

1.	A	5.	E	9.	D
2.	C	6.	D	10.	B
3.	B	7.	E		
4.	A	8.	C		

LABORATORY EXERCISE 11
Supplemental Radiographic Techniques and Tips

1.	B	5.	B	9.	C
2.	A	6.	A	10.	D
3.	C	7.	B		
4.	C	8.	D		

LABORATORY EXERCISE 12
Panoramic Radiographic Technique

1.	A	4.	D	7.	B
2.	D	5.	B	8.	D
3.	C	6.	A	9.	D

10. Essay—See outline for key points to be included in this answer.

LABORATORY EXERCISE 13
Radiographic Quality Assurance

1.	C	5.	A	9.	D
2.	D	6.	C	10.	A
3.	A	7.	B		
4.	B	8.	B		

LABORATORY EXERCISE 14
Radiographic Interpretation

1.	C	5.	D	9.	D
2.	A	6.	C	10.	B
3.	C	7.	D		
4.	A	8.	B		